12/14   SIT

Books should be returned or renewed by the last date above. Renew by phone 08458 247 200 or online www.kent.gov.uk/libs

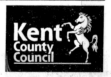

Libraries & Archives

CUSTOMER
SERVICE
EXCELLENCE
UK
The Government Standard

this role he oversees a global network of programmes to promote improved care and education for people with diabetes as well as prevention of type 2 diabetes.

Dedicated to the memory of
Tony Cavan

Reverse
your
Diabetes

The Step-by-Step Plan to Take
Control of Type 2 Diabetes

DR DAVID CAVAN

LONDON

1 3 5 7 9 10 8 6 4 2

Vermilion, an imprint of Ebury Publishing,
20 Vauxhall Bridge Road,
London SW1V 2SA

Vermilion is part of the Penguin Random House group of companies whose
addresses can be found at global.penguinrandomhouse.com

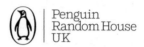
Penguin
Random House
UK

First published by Vermilion in 2014

www.eburypublishing.co.uk

A CIP catalogue record for this book is available from the British Library

ISBN 9780091948252

Designed and set by seagulls.net
Printed and bound by CPI Group (UK) Ltd, Croydon CR0 4YY

Penguin Random House is committed to a sustainable future for our
business, our readers and our planet. This book is made from
Forest Stewardship Council® certified paper.

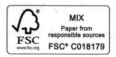

CONTENTS

PREFACE

I have worked as a diabetes specialist for many years. Very early on, I came to realise that the vast majority of diabetes management is done by the person with diabetes, and therefore it is essential that everyone with diabetes is given the appropriate training and education that will enable them to manage their diabetes as well as possible.

From 1996 until 2013, I worked as a consultant at the Bournemouth Diabetes and Endocrine Centre. During that time I developed my interest in patient education and launched a self-management programme for people with type 1 diabetes called BERTIE. I also helped develop an education programme for people with type 2 diabetes called 'Focus on Diabetes'. Focus had been started originally in 1993 and in its time was quite radical – providing high-quality education to people at the time of diagnosis with type 2 diabetes as part of their routine care. The programme continues, in a different form, to this day. The key message of the programme was to encourage people to change their lifestyles. Many did, and as a result their diabetes control improved dramatically – and quickly too. However, after a few years it became apparent that the improvements we saw began to disappear and at this stage it would be common to start them on tablets to help control their diabetes.

During the early years of this century the emphasis shifted to using medication to achieve as near-normal levels of blood glucose as possible; in more and more cases this would include the use of insulin. Initially this led to good improvements in diabetes control, but over time I could see that many people were beginning to put on weight, and once again the improvements would reverse. As I will describe in the book, a number of new medications have been introduced over the past 10 years. Each one came full of promise and, like insulin, often led to temporary improvements. But over time their effects diminished – and in some cases the drugs have been withdrawn because of safety concerns.

I now began to question the medical training I had received that had focused so much attention on medication as the best way of controlling type 2 diabetes. I also began to question the standard dietary advice for people with diabetes, namely to base all meals on carbohydrates. As all carbohydrates are broken down in the body into glucose it seemed an illogical way to keep blood glucose levels under control. I followed the experiences of people with diabetes who contributed to Internet chat forums (such as diabetes.co.uk and diabetes-support.org.uk) and increasingly came to understand the concerns many held about the treatment they were receiving using established medical and dietary practice. In 2011 I began to suggest to people with type 2 diabetes that rather than increase their medication they could try reducing their carbohydrate intake instead. And in many cases it worked. Over the next year I began to recommend this as the preferred option, and saw many people gain good control of their diabetes – including some who came off insulin altogether after many years of injecting.

This certainly challenged the conventional wisdom that type 2 diabetes is a progressive disease that, over time, will likely require long-term treatment with insulin. The realisation that people could actually come off insulin if they changed their diet suggested to me that what they were eating had a far more powerful effect on their diabetes than any medication. It also was consistent with newly emerging research-based evidence that type 2 diabetes can actually be reversed. These results initially came from people with diabetes who had weight-loss surgery and afterwards no longer had diabetes. Others, who had lost weight by other means, also were able to reverse their diabetes.

This in turn has led to a greater understanding about the nature of type 2 diabetes: far from being a progressive one-way street we now understand that the progression of diabetes can be halted, and even reversed, by dietary changes. This is because the accumulation of fat in the body appears to be directly responsible for at least some of the changes that occur in diabetes – namely insulin resistance (that is, insulin not working properly), high blood glucose levels and weight gain. Losing weight leads to loss of fat from the body, lower glucose levels and less insulin resistance.

I firmly believe that this profound change in our understanding about type 2 diabetes should be shared with everyone who has the condition. It represents a change from a message of despair (where deterioration and complications are inevitable) to one of hope that the condition can be reversed.

Therefore I have written this book to provide people with type 2 diabetes with information to make changes that will maximise each person's ability to reverse the diabetes disease process. For some this will mean they no longer have diabetes, for some it will mean they have much better control of their diabetes through diet changes alone, and for others that they have better control of their diabetes on less medication. So while the first group will have reversed their diabetes completely to normal glucose metabolism (which is called 'remission'), others will have partially reversed their diabetes to varying extents, and as a result will have improved their current and future health.

In my current role at the International Diabetes Federation I am aware of the massive global health and economic threat type 2 diabetes poses. The fact that type 2 diabetes can be reversed provides a message of hope at national level, as even wealthy countries will soon find it very difficult to afford the health care and economic costs of such a large percentage of their population having diabetes.

Dr David Cavan

June 2014

CHAPTER 1

FIRST OF ALL: DO NOT WORRY, TAKE CONTROL

If you have recently been diagnosed with type 2 diabetes then this book is designed just for you. Its aim is to help you learn how best to manage the condition, and possibly even to reverse it. It is based on over 20 years' direct experience in managing people with type 2 diabetes, from the time of diagnosis right through to those who have had the condition for decades – most of whom are still very much alive and kicking. It is not a medical textbook, nor an airy-fairy self-help book, but a book that is designed to give you the practical tools and the support and encouragement you need in order to take control of your diabetes – along with a good measure of hope for the future.

If you have had type 2 diabetes for 20 years or more – well done, you have managed your condition at a time when the tools available were considerably fewer than they are today. However, you were probably told that diabetes is irreversible, and over time will likely get worse. By reading this book, you will learn that this doesn't have to be the case, and will find some new things that you can try to help you better manage your diabetes.

It is well recognised that things that happen around the time of diagnosis – both good and bad – can have a long-lasting effect. So the better you can deal with the diagnosis, the quicker you can take control of your diabetes, and the quicker you deal with any negative issues surrounding the diagnosis, the better the outlook for the future.

So, if you have recently developed type 2 diabetes, how does this make you feel? Before doing anything else, it is worth pausing to consider this so that you can address any feelings you may experience that might get in the way of you being able to take control of the condition now and in the future. People can experience a whole range of feelings when they are diagnosed with type 2 diabetes, including relief that they know what was causing troublesome symptoms, guilt that they may have eaten too much of the wrong things, anger that it should affect them, fear for the future, loneliness and a whole host of other feelings and emotions.

Such feelings are completely natural and it is good to acknowledge them and, if possible, to talk about them with someone close to you, someone sympathetic who is able to listen even if they don't have the answers to the many questions you may well have.

The reason for discussing this right at the beginning is not just to be 'touchy-feely', but to acknowledge that if certain emotions are not properly addressed they can have a massive effect on physical and mental health for years to come. It is better to confront your fears and worries so you can discover – through your own research or others' personal experience – the tools to address these concerns, and hopefully put them behind you. There are a number of websites, which include discussion forums where you can share your feelings with others who have been through the same experience. Some of these are listed in appendix 1.

The point I want to make at the outset is that whatever your own situation I would encourage you not to worry or to be fearful. Our medical understanding of type 2 diabetes and its management has changed beyond all recognition in the past 20 years, and we are learning more all the time. Our ability to control diabetes has never been better and we now know that in some situations it is possible to reverse type 2 diabetes. As a result of these medical advances, the risk of incurring disabling complications of the disease has reduced significantly.

In addition there are now education programmes available in many parts of the country where you can learn how to take control of your diabetes and how to protect your long-term health. There are some steps that you can take immediately that will help reduce your glucose levels, get you feeling better and set you on the path to taking control of your diabetes. I call this my diabetes 'first aid' guide – simple steps that anyone can take. You may not feel that they all apply to you, but I would encourage you to look at the list below and choose one or two changes that you feel you could make immediately:

FIRST AID GUIDE TO TAKING CONTROL OF TYPE 2 DIABETES

Drink

1. Stop using sugar in tea or coffee (use sweeteners if necessary).
2. Drink plenty of water and avoid sweet drinks such as fruit juice, smoothies, squashes and fizzy drinks (use sugar-free drinks as far as possible).
3. Try to cut down the amount of alcohol you drink, especially drinks containing carbohydrate such as beer, cider or sweet wines.

Food

1. Try to avoid sweet foods such as cakes, biscuits, jam, sweets or chocolate except as an occasional treat.
2. Try to eat less potatoes, rice, pasta and bread.

3. Try to eat more fresh vegetables and fresh fruit such as apples, pears and tangerines (one piece of fruit at a time).
4. Try to cut down the size of your usual food portions.

Exercise
1. Try to take a 15-minute walk every day.
2. Use stairs instead of lifts or escalators.
3. Walk or cycle instead of using the car or bus for short journeys.

These tips reflect the key elements of managing type 2 diabetes in the short term: eating less sugar and starchy food and becoming more active. We will cover these in more detail later in the book, but making these changes now will make a big difference to most people newly diagnosed with type 2 diabetes. However, please note that nothing is banned! Where food is concerned, the message is 'try to cut down', rather than 'stop altogether'. If you really enjoy chocolate, you will do much better by learning to have a small amount occasionally than trying to stop eating chocolate ever again. That is more likely to lead to resentment, temptation to eat 'forbidden fruit', and levels of guilt afterwards. Resentment, temptation and guilt are three negative emotions to try to avoid for good mental health!

So please do try and make some changes, however small, as suggested in the box. If you do not feel you can make any changes right now, you may wish to set yourself a goal of one change you feel you could realistically make in the next two weeks. Please do not wait until you 'know it all' before making a start. Any changes you make now can be fine-tuned at any time as you go along.

As you make changes, you will hopefully begin to see some improvements in your blood glucose levels, your feeling of well-being or your weight – and possibly all three. Taking control of your diabetes in this way will be the first step towards reversing your diabetes. We will discuss what we mean by this later in the book, but for now the message is that anything you can do to reduce your weight and your blood glucose levels by making changes to your lifestyle (diet and exercise) will be the beginning of the process of reversing the changes in your body that have led to your diagnosis of type 2 diabetes. Some people will be able to reverse their diabetes completely, so that they no longer have diabetes. Others will make some progress in the right direction, but will still have diabetes. The bottom line is that anything that leads to a more normal body weight and lower blood glucose levels will lead to a healthier future.

The message of this first chapter is 'do not worry, take control' and I hope that the little I have said so far will provide some reassurance. However, it may be that you have specific reasons to feel very worried – because of symptoms you may be experiencing, or because of other problems which might be causing anxiety or depression. If you feel this applies to you, visit your GP and ask for help.

CHAPTER 2

WHAT IS TYPE 2 DIABETES?

A HISTORY OF DIABETES

The full name of the condition is diabetes mellitus, which literally means, 'passing (perhaps more accurately "pissing") honey' since the condition results in the urine containing glucose and tasting sweet. Diabetes was described in ancient Egypt, in the Papyrus Ebers that date from around 1500BC, as a disease where urine is too plentiful. Susrata of the Hindus wrote in 1000BC that the urine was sweet and that ants and flies were attracted to it. He thought that diabetes was a disease of the urinary tract (kidneys and bladder) and wrote that it could be inherited or develop as a result of dietary excess or obesity (perhaps referring to type 1 and type 2 diabetes respectively). The recommended treatment was exercise. It was not until the 17th century that it was discovered that the urine was sweet because it contained sugar and that diabetes was a disease of the pancreas rather than the kidneys. This was discovered in 1682 by Swiss anatomist Johan Brunner (1653–1727) who removed the pancreas from dogs and found that this led to diabetes. In 1797, the Scottish military surgeon John Rollo heated the urine of patients until a sugary cake was all that remained. He noted that the volume of the cake increased if the patient ate bread, grains and fruit (high in carbohydrate), but decreased if he or she ate meat and poultry (low carbohydrate). He described the case of a Captain Meredith who took to a diet low in carbohydrate and high in fat and protein. His weight fell from 16st 8lbs (105kg) to 11st 8lbs (73.5kg) and his health improved. At the time diabetes was reported as being relatively rare and associated with wealth.

It was not until the end of the 19th century that the role of insulin became apparent. In 1889 two German physicians Joseph von Mehring (1849–1908) and Oskar Minkowski (1858–1931) working jointly at the University of Strasbourg removed the pancreas from dogs. They noticed that this caused the unfortunate animals to urinate frequently on the floor – despite being previously house-trained. Testing the urine they found high levels of sugar, thus confirming the link between the pancreas and diabetes. This was then reversed by the transplantation of small pieces of the pancreas back into the dog's abdomen. Incidentally, since 1966 the Minkowski Prize has been awarded annually by the European Association for the Study of Diabetes (EASD) to recognise research that has contributed to the advancement of knowledge concerning diabetes. The recipient is invited to deliver the Minkowski Lecture at the annual EASD conference.

In 1921 Canadian medical scientist (and future Nobel laureate) Sir Frederick Grant Banting (1891–1941) and Dr Charles Best (1899–1978) isolated an extract of pancreatic islets of Langerhans cells and found this reduced glucose levels in diabetic dogs. The following year this extract (a prototype of insulin) was injected for the first time into a patient with diabetes – a 14-year-old boy called Leonard Thompson.

Piece by piece, the puzzle was being completed, and by the 1920s it was established that diabetes is characterised by an excess of sugar (glucose) in the blood resulting in the glucose excess found in the urine. The disease was often seen in overweight people in whom it could be controlled by the patient adopting a low-carbohydrate diet. In other patients, insulin, extracted from animal pancreases and given by injection, led to a fall in blood glucose levels.

TYPES OF DIABETES

By the 1970s it had become clear that there were two distinct types of diabetes:

1. Type 1 diabetes usually occurs first in children or young adults. It comes on quite suddenly with marked

symptoms such as thirst and weight loss, and can only be treated by insulin injections.

2. Type 2 diabetes usually occurs in later life and it has become increasingly clear that it is related to increasing weight as a result of excess food intake and/or too little exercise. Its onset is usually far more gradual, without any specific symptoms, and is sometimes first diagnosed by a screening blood test. Type 2 diabetes can be controlled by lifestyle changes, principally by modifying diet. Many people are prescribed drugs to control type 2 diabetes, and until relatively recently it was thought that most people would eventually need insulin.

Since then our understanding has developed further: there are rare forms of type 2 diabetes that occur in young people (so called maturity-onset diabetes of the young or MODY). These are inherited conditions, are not associated with weight gain, and there is usually a strong family history of diabetes. Although they usually present in childhood, most cases can be controlled with tablets rather than insulin.

It has also become apparent that the distinction between type 1 and type 2 diabetes is not as clear-cut as previously thought, and for people who are diagnosed in their forties and fifties, there may be a period of uncertainty before one can definitely distinguish between the two. For example, some overweight adults present quite acutely with very high glucose levels and require insulin at diagnosis, but can later be switched to tablets. Conversely, there is a type of type 1 diabetes that occurs in older people, sometimes referred to as LADA – latent autoimmune diabetes of adulthood. Like type 1 diabetes, people with this condition are not overweight, though the onset is more like type 2 diabetes, and they may be treated with tablets for a period. However, within a few years it becomes clear they need insulin, and from that time they behave very much like type 1 diabetes sufferers.

Gestational diabetes is a condition in which diabetes occurs during pregnancy. It is similar to type 2 diabetes and can be controlled with diet in some cases, otherwise insulin is used as tablets are generally not advised during pregnancy. It usually reverses once the baby is born, but the mother is at increased risk of developing type 2 diabetes in later life.

Diabetes can also arise as a result of other diseases affecting hormones (e.g. acromegaly which is a condition caused by the presence of too much growth hormone, or Cushing's disease, which is caused by the presence of too much steroid hormone, cortisol). These cases generally reverse once the underlying condition has been treated. Cortisol is the body's natural steroid, and people who have been treated with steroids for long periods of time for conditions such as asthma may develop diabetes. Diabetes also occurs if other diseases affect the pancreas or if the pancreas has been wholly or partly removed.

While some parts of this book may be helpful to people with other types of diabetes, it is intended specifically to help people with type 2 diabetes learn how to manage their condition. The rest of this book refers solely to type 2 diabetes.

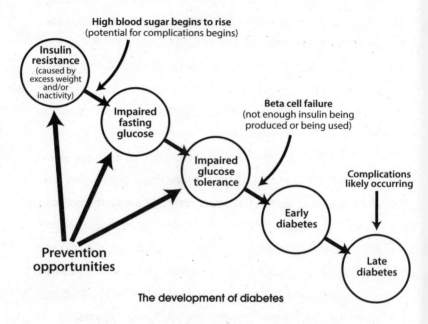

The development of diabetes

MAKING A DIAGNOSIS OF DIABETES

The typical symptoms of diabetes include excessive urination, excessive thirst, tiredness, blurred vision, weight loss, and infections such as thrush. These arise as follows: in diabetes, glucose cannot enter the body's cells and so it accumulates in the bloodstream. As glucose (a carbohydrate that is used by cells as a source of energy) is not getting into the body's cells, they are starved of energy and this leads to weight loss and tiredness. As the blood glucose rises the kidneys try to excrete the excess glucose in the urine. This explains why glucose can be detected in the urine and its sugary nature provides an ideal environment for the growth of bacteria and fungi, which leads to urinary infections and thrush (candidiasis). In order to excrete glucose, the kidneys need to excrete a larger volume of water (otherwise you would be peeing out sugar lumps) and this leads to dehydration, which in turn leads to excessive thirst. High glucose levels in the eyes leads to blurred vision.

In many cases of type 2 diabetes, people are diagnosed with no or only very mild symptoms. This is because diabetes is being picked up very early as a result of screening blood tests arranged by GPs in people who do not yet have any symptoms of the disease. In other cases, people may have had diabetes for some time, which has not been diagnosed. In these cases, blood glucose levels may rise high enough for some of these symptoms to occur.

Diabetes is diagnosed by blood tests. This means that if you have symptoms that you think may be due to diabetes but the blood tests are normal, you do not have diabetes. On the other hand if your blood tests are diagnostic of diabetes, then you have diabetes, even if you do not have any symptoms.

Diabetes can be diagnosed by a measurement of random blood glucose, fasting blood glucose, by a glucose tolerance test (see page 17) or by an HbA1c test (see page 18).

1. Random blood glucose

This is often the first test that will be done and can be performed at any time of the day after breakfast. The result is expressed as the amount of glucose molecules per litre of blood and interpreted as follows:

Random blood glucose level	Interpretation
Up to 7.7mmol/l	Normal
7.8 to 11.1mmol/l	Impaired glucose tolerance (IGT)
11.1mmol/l or above	Diabetes

If the random glucose is normal it is unlikely that the person has diabetes; however, if it is in the impaired glucose tolerance range, then a fasting glucose or a glucose tolerance test will usually be performed (see opposite).

2. Fasting blood glucose

This is a blood test taken after a fast of 12 hours, during which time only water can be taken. The test is generally performed first thing in the morning. The results are expressed as the amount of glucose molecules per litre of blood and are interpreted as follows:

Fasting blood glucose level	Interpretation
Up to 6.0mmol/l	Normal
6.1 to 7.0mmol/l	Impaired fasting hyperglycaemia
7.0mmol/l or above	Diabetes

If both the fasting and random glucose levels are normal, then the patient does not have diabetes.

3. **Glucose tolerance test**
   This is a standardised test where a fasting glucose level is measured and then the patient is asked to drink a liquid (such as Lucozade) that contains 75g of glucose. A further blood test is taken two hours after the drink to see how high the glucose level has risen. The results are interpreted in the same way as the fasting and random tests above. If either the fasting *or* the two-hour values are diagnostic, then the patient has diabetes. Both have to be normal to exclude the diagnosis.

4. **Glycated haemoglobin**
   When the level of blood glucose is higher than normal, the excess glucose attaches to a number of different molecules in the body. For example when glucose attaches to the lens of the eye, it can lead to the development of cataracts, or if it attaches to soft tissue in the shoulder it may lead to a frozen shoulder. This process of attachment is termed glycation. Red blood cells contain haemoglobin, which is the substance that carries oxygen in the blood cells to the different tissues around the body and gives blood its red colour. A small amount of haemoglobin in each blood cell is glycated and just how much will depend on the amount of glucose present in the bloodstream. Red blood cells last for about four months before they are

'recycled', and the amount of glycated haemoglobin in any one cell gradually increases over this time. Blood glucose levels change constantly according to food intake and activity levels, and so a single measurement is of little use in monitoring diabetic control. Glycated haemoglobin (abbreviated as HbA1c), on the other hand, is used to assess glucose levels over a longer period of time, and for many years has been the gold standard means of assessing diabetic control (see chapter 9). Recently, it has also been introduced as a means of diagnosing type 2 diabetes. Its measurement involves a simple blood test that can be taken at any time of day (as it reflects glucose control over the past 6–8 weeks). Historically, HbA1c was expressed as the percentage of haemoglobin that was glycated. In 2011, a new system if units was introduced, which expresses the glycated component as a concentration of the total haemoglobin (mmol/mol). However, many people still refer to the old units. Furthermore, in many other countries, and in much international literature, the new units haven't caught on at all. I will therefore present both units in this book. In people without diabetes, glycated haemoglobin is generally below 40mmol/mol (5.5 per cent). A measurement of 48mmol/mol (6.5 per cent) or above is considered diagnostic of type 2 diabetes. However, it is important to be aware that a level below this does not rule out diabetes, and if there is any doubt then a glucose tolerance test should be performed.

You will notice that for the blood glucose tests, there is a middle category, which is higher than normal, but not yet diagnostic of diabetes. Impaired fasting hyperglycaemia and impaired glucose tolerance both represent a pre-diabetes state that will likely progress to diabetes. It is important to be aware that these diagnostic numbers are arbitrary numbers that have been chosen to make the diagnosis of diabetes straightforward. Given that the disease process that leads to diabetes is not an on/off process, but a gradual deterioration in the body's ability to handle glucose, then I would strongly advise anyone who finds they are in these middle categories to adopt the lifestyle changes recommended in this book, as they can help reverse the situation (as explained in more detail in chapter 6).

THE ROLE OF INSULIN IN KEEPING GLUCOSE LEVELS UNDER CONTROL

In order to understand why glucose levels rise in people with diabetes, it is important to understand how insulin controls glucose levels when everything is working normally.

Glucose is a type of sugar that is used for energy by nearly all types of cells in the body and it is essential that all parts of the body have a steady supply of glucose. This glucose is obtained from the food we eat: all carbohydrates (sugars and starch) that we eat are broken down into glucose, which is then absorbed from the gut into the bloodstream so that it can be carried to all tissues and used as energy. Any spare glucose is taken up into the muscles and liver where it is stored in the form of glycogen. Glycogen in the muscles is then available for later use if the muscles need extra energy (e.g. during intensive exercise). Once the glycogen stores are full, any excess glucose is converted to fat and stored in the liver.

While glucose only enters the body when we eat or drink, the body's cells require a constant supply of glucose in order to function properly. The liver, which releases some of its stored glucose into the bloodstream, provides this service and ensures that just the right amount of glucose is available during periods when we are not eating (overnight, for example). In a person without diabetes the amount of glucose in the bloodstream is kept at around 4–6mmol per litre.

The level of glucose in the bloodstream is controlled by insulin. Insulin is a hormone that is produced by the pancreas. The pancreas is an organ that sits just below the ribcage, behind the stomach. Like many of the body's organs, the pancreas does a lot of different things. However, it has two main functions: one is to produce enzymes that are released directly into the small intestine in order to break down food so it can be absorbed into the bloodstream. These enzymes include amylase, which breaks down starch into glucose; lipase, which breaks down fat, and protease, which breaks down proteins.

The other main function of the pancreas is to produce hormones. These are chemicals that are released into the bloodstream and which have effects all around the body. Insulin is one of the hormones produced by the pancreas, and its job is to regulate the amount of glucose in the bloodstream, ensuring that cells get the right amount of glucose at all times. It does this in a number of ways:

1. When we eat a meal the carbohydrate in the meal is converted into glucose in the gut and passes through the gut wall into the bloodstream. The body detects that the glucose level in the blood is rising and this leads to the pancreas producing additional insulin.

2. This insulin acts on individual cells to allow glucose to enter them. Insulin molecules attach to a receptor on the cell membrane that opens up to allow glucose in. Insulin is often likened to a 'key' that opens the cell's 'door' allowing glucose to enter the cell.

3. Insulin also stops the liver and muscles from releasing stored glucose into the blood; this allows spare glucose to be added to the glycogen stores.

4. When we are not eating, the pancreas continually produces a small amount of insulin that controls the release of glucose from the liver. In the liver insulin acts like a tap that turns off the release of glucose from the liver. If glucose levels in the blood drop too low then less insulin will be produced (opening the tap) allowing more glucose to be released from the liver.

On the other hand, if glucose levels rise then more insulin is produced, closing the tap and slowing down the release of glucose from the liver.

The main problem in type 2 diabetes is that insulin doesn't work very well; this reduced effectiveness interferes with both the action of insulin in turning off the tap that releases glucose stored in the liver into the bloodstream and its role in opening the cell doors to allow glucose to enter the body's cells after a meal.

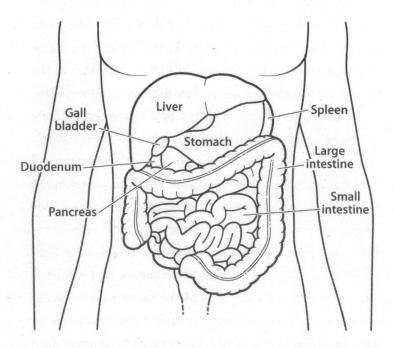

It seems that the problem starts in the liver that becomes 'immune' or resistant to the effect of insulin – so that even when insulin is present, the liver keeps releasing glucose into the bloodstream. This is called 'insulin resistance' and to try to get round this, the pancreas produces more and more insulin in an attempt to control the release of glucose from the liver. For a while this may work in keeping the blood glucose level under control, but eventually the liver becomes resistant to even these high levels of insulin, and the level of glucose in the blood rises. Diabetes develops once the blood glucose rises above a certain level – that is above 7mmol per litre if fasting, or above 11.1mmol/l after a meal.

The progression of type 2 diabetes after diagnosis was perhaps best documented in the United Kingdom Prospective Diabetes Study (UKPDS)[1] that studied the progress of people with diabetes diagnosed in the 1970s. This showed that even with the best treatment available at the time, glucose (and HbA1c) levels rose progressively over the years following diagnosis. Blood pressure and cholesterol levels were also high, and this study emphasised that type 2 diabetes is not just a glucose disorder, but also one in which blood pressure and cholesterol levels can cause problems. This is actually not surprising as high insulin levels have an effect on retaining sodium (salt) in the body that leads to high blood pressure. Insulin resistance is also associated with high cholesterol levels, and high glucose levels are associated with another type of body fat, called triglycerides. In approaching the management of type 2 diabetes it is therefore important to monitor not just glucose levels, but also blood pressure and cholesterol, and where possible use strategies which will reduce rather than increase insulin levels.

THE BLURRED BOUNDARY BETWEEN TYPE 1 AND TYPE 2 DIABETES

Earlier in this chapter we learnt that the distinction between type 1 and type 2 diabetes is not as clear-cut as was once thought and several different 'types' of type 2 diabetes have now been identified. The diagnosis of type 1 or type 2 diabetes is usually done clinically, that is according to the symptoms and signs present at the time of diagnosis rather than by any formal testing. The reason for this is that there is no readily available test that will say for definite whether a patient has type 1 diabetes or type 2 diabetes. The nearest we have are tests to check the levels of different antibodies to the islet cells that are present in many, but not all, people with type 1 diabetes. If these antibodies are present in the bloodstream it is very likely the person has type 1 diabetes. However, if they are not found the individual may still have type 1 diabetes. The other test that can be performed is to check the level of C-peptide in the blood. C-peptide is a by-product of the production of insulin, and for every molecule of insulin produced in the pancreas, one molecule of C-peptide is also produced. It is uncertain whether C-peptide has any biological effect, but it is very useful as a marker of insulin production. So, if it is found in the blood, it means that insulin is being produced and the person is therefore likely to have type 2 diabetes. This information has to be used with caution as many people with type 1 diabetes continue to produce insulin for up to two years (during the honeymoon period), and there is now evidence that some insulin production may last for up to five years.

There is also the matter of ketones. Ketones are substances found in the blood that result from the breakdown of fat. When the body cannot produce insulin (that enables or facilitates the use of glucose by the body's cells for energy) then fat is broken down for the necessary energy instead, and this in turn produces ketones. At high levels ketones can cause the blood to become acidic, and this is the basis of the condition known as diabetic ketoacidosis, which is a potentially very serious condition in people with type 1 diabetes. The level of ketones in the blood can be tested for using a special meter and test strips, similar to those used to test blood glucose. However, in most cases a urine test (using a ketone test strip) is performed to check for evidence of ketone production. A small amount of ketones will be present in the urine of someone who has not eaten for several hours, but higher levels of ketones in someone with diabetes generally mean that they are deficient in insulin, and need insulin treatment.

It was generally thought that if a person had ketones in their urine (or blood) at the time they were diagnosed with diabetes it meant they had type 1 diabetes. They would then be started on insulin and told they would need insulin treatment for life. Over recent years, however, it has become apparent that some people labelled, in all good faith, as having type 1 diabetes do not actually have it. I have particularly seen this in some patients who are overweight and who 'look' as if they have type 2 diabetes. When tested they have C-peptide in their blood, demonstrating that they are producing insulin, and, in some cases, it has been possible for them to stop insulin treatment altogether.

This suggests that people with type 2 diabetes may also produce ketones, especially at diagnosis and during periods of illness, and we should therefore guard against labelling someone as having type 1 diabetes on the basis of ketones present at diagnosis. In fairness to doctors and nurses the ambiguities of the various tests can make it very difficult to make an accurate diagnosis when someone first develops diabetes and it is entirely appropriate to start insulin if someone has ketones or their glucose levels are very high (as will be discussed in more detail in chapter 14). However, unless there is clear-cut evidence of type 1 diabetes, such as presenting with ketoacidosis or positive antibodies, it is entirely reasonable to review treatments, especially in patients who are overweight or require high doses of insulin (e.g. over 90 units a day). This is particularly important given our new understanding that type 2 diabetes can be reversed and it should also lead us to rethink our approach to people started on insulin in the past in the belief that they had type 1 diabetes.

Similarly people who are diagnosed with type 2 diabetes and who are initially treated with tablets and then moved on to insulin may find that with appropriate lifestyle changes they can come off insulin. Again, this is in contrast to what they would have been told in the past that once you need insulin, you need it for life.

The significance of this is that a number of people currently on insulin believe there is no option to insulin treatment whereas, in the light of our current understanding, there very well may be. With appropriate lifestyle changes as described in the following chapters it should certainly be possible for many people to reduce the amount of insulin they need, and for some to come off it altogether while still keeping their diabetes under control.

In summary:

▶ you were overweight at the time of diagnosis and are still overweight (i.e. you have a BMI above 27)
▶ you require over 90 units of insulin a day
▶ you have no history of diabetic ketoacidosis

It is very important that any changes to your diabetes treatment are made in consultation with your doctor, as it is dangerous to stop insulin if you do happen to have type 1 diabetes.

CHAPTER 3

THE COMPLICATIONS OF DIABETES

The term 'complications of diabetes' generally refers to the long-term effects that diabetes has on various parts of the body. At their worst these can lead to blindness, kidney failure and amputations. It is a sad fact that many people will have experience of relatives and friends with diabetes who have been affected in this way. Others will have heard (well-meaning) friends tell of the person they know who has become blind and lost both legs as a result of diabetes. On hearing such stories it is understandable for someone recently diagnosed with diabetes to become overly fatalistic about the future, and fail to put in the necessary effort to control diabetes on the mistaken assumption that significant complications are inevitable.

However, even if type 2 diabetes is an inevitably progressive disease (and in chapter 6 we will learn that this is not necessarily the case) such complications themselves are by no means inevitable – especially for someone who is newly diagnosed. In fact with good management, it is safe to say that the more severe complications can be avoided altogether, and milder ones that might occur can be treated or controlled, ensuring they do not cause any problems. This is because the risk of complications is directly related to the level of glucose in the bloodstream, usually assessed by the blood test called HbA1c (see chapter 2). Simply put, the higher the HbA1c, the greater the risk. Keeping glucose levels as normal as possible (equivalent to an HbA1c between 40 and 50mmol/l or roughly 6 to 7 per cent) greatly minimises the risk of complications.

The key to good management is lifestyle changes, with or without the use of medication, right from the time of diagnosis. This is why I consider it vitally important that at diagnosis people have the opportunity to learn how best to manage their diabetes; there is good evidence that the gains made in the early days and weeks from diagnosis lead to lasting health benefits. In the past it was not unusual for people to have type 2 diabetes for many years before they were diagnosed, perhaps because the symptoms were initially quite mild or they did not feel unwell enough to visit their doctor. As a result people could already have evidence of advanced complications of diabetes by the time they were diagnosed. Fortunately this is becoming an increasingly rare situation as more people are aware about the nature, and rising incidence, of diabetes, and GPs have become very good at testing people who are at risk of developing diabetes.

In this chapter I will discuss the main complications of diabetes, but my main emphasis will be on what measures can be taken, both by you as someone with diabetes and your doctor to prevent them.

As I have already stated, complications arise as a result of the effect of high blood glucose levels on the body. It is estimated that it takes at least 10 years for advanced complications to become established, and so a few weeks or months of high glucose levels are unlikely to lead to lasting damage. It is in the cases where glucose levels have been high for years that the risk of complications are seen at their greatest. And whereas type 2 diabetes was originally seen mainly as a 'sugar disease', the UKPDS has shown us that high blood pressure and high cholesterol levels are also major risk factors in the development of complications. As people with diabetes tend to have higher blood pressure and cholesterol levels than people without diabetes, keeping both under good control is as important as managing blood glucose levels.

DAMAGE TO LARGE BLOOD VESSELS – VASCULAR DISEASE

Most of the complications of diabetes are due to damage to blood vessels, known as vascular disease. Blood vessels are commonly divided into large and small blood vessels. Large blood vessels are the tubes that carry blood from the heart to all parts of the body (the arteries) and back from the various parts of the body to the heart (the veins). The heart pumps constantly to maintain blood pressure and to keep blood flowing through the system. As the arteries reach out across the body they divide into smaller and smaller branches until they form very small blood vessels called capillaries. It is here that the nutrients contained within the blood (such as oxygen and glucose) leave the blood vessels and enter the surrounding tissues, where they are used as energy by the cells within the tissue (e.g. a muscle). It is a bit like a domestic central heating system where the heart is like the boiler (creating the pressure), the blood vessels are like the copper pipes (carrying the hot water around) and the radiators are a bit like the capillaries (where the energy is transferred to heat the air). However, the analogy then begins to break down as in the body capillaries also collect waste products such as carbon dioxide from the tissues to be recycled. Household radiators don't do that, yet.

However, just as the pipes in the central heating system can get furred up, leaky or blocked, so can the blood vessels. When we are born our blood vessels are beautifully smooth and clean inside, but as we grow older the insides of our blood vessels start to fur up with cholesterol and other substances that form atheroma, so-called narrowing of the arteries. If the narrowing becomes critical then the part of the body supplied by that blood vessel will be deprived of oxygen and other essential nutrients. At the point when a blood vessel becomes completely blocked the tissue it supplies will be damaged, and part of it may die to be replaced by scar tissue. If this occurs in a coronary artery in the heart, it is referred to as a heart attack; in the brain it is called a stroke. Blockage of an artery in the leg may lead to tissue damage in the foot. The underlying process is the same, but the effect depends on which artery is affected and what part of the body it serves.

Now of course you will be aware that heart attacks and strokes occur not only in people with diabetes and are actually quite common in our society. There are a number of factors that increase the risk of these sorts of serious health problems, including smoking, having a family history of such diseases, having high blood pressure or a high cholesterol level and being overweight. Type 2 diabetes is described by some doctors as being part of the 'metabolic syndrome'. This is a group of conditions that are often found together and includes diabetes, obesity, high blood pressure and high cholesterol levels. There is evidence that insulin resistance (as described in chapter 2) directly leads to high blood pressure and cholesterol levels, and it is quite possible that this is the main problem in the metabolic syndrome. Regardless of the precise cause, the fact that blood pressure and cholesterol levels tend to be higher in people with diabetes explains why problems such as heart attacks, foot disease and strokes have been more common in people with diabetes.

Now, there is not much you can do about your family history and if you have high blood pressure or high cholesterol this may also be partly due to the genes you have inherited from your parents. However, effective treatments are available to treat high blood pressure or cholesterol (see chapter 16) and everyone can try to stop smoking and lose some weight – and if successful, will significantly reduce the risk of vascular disease, even in people with diabetes.

Whereas large blood vessel diseases can occur in people without diabetes, small blood vessel disease is more specific to diabetes. This is because it generally results directly from the excess of glucose in the bloodstream. Over time this excess causes small blood vessels (capillaries) to become blocked or to become leaky. While this process will occur to some extent all over the body, its main effects are seen in two critical areas – the eyes and the kidneys.

DIABETIC EYE DISEASE – RETINOPATHY

Diabetic eye disease (known as retinopathy) is probably the most common complication of diabetes, and also the most studied. This is because it is possible directly to see and document the damage to the blood vessels. Below is a photograph taken of the back of the eye through the pupil. It shows the retina, the lining of cells inside the back of the eye, which is orange in colour. The capillaries fan out from the optic disc to supply blood to all parts of the retina. These are seen as smooth fine red lines. After many years of high glucose levels these capillaries can become irregular (leaving tiny red dots poking through the surface) or begin to leak (leaving red or white blots). This is so-called background diabetic retinopathy, and does not affect eyesight. Over time, however, damage to a capillary can cause the area of retina it serves to be starved of oxygen and glucose, and this can change the appearance of the retina. This stage, known as pre-proliferative retinopathy, does not adversely affect eyesight either.

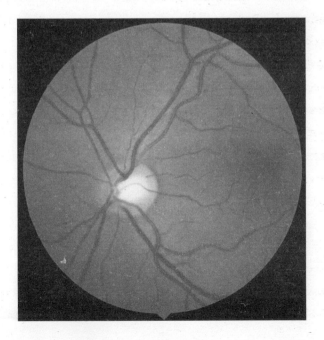

There are two types of retinopathy that do affect vision. The first is a progression of the process described above, where the damaged retina sends out signals to stimulate the formation of new blood vessels to supply the area covered by the defective capillary. This may seem like a good thing, but unfortunately these new capillaries have a tendency to grow forwards into the vitreous (the jelly that fills the eyeball) and they are also very fragile, which means they have a tendency to bleed into the eyeball, and it is this that can cause blindness.

The other type of sight-threatening retinopathy is maculopathy. This is where the earlier stage of retinopathy affects the central part of the retina, the macula. As this area is used for central vision, any damage will affect one's ability to focus on what one is looking at. This will make it difficult to read, or drive a car, for example, even though the surrounding areas of retina may be relatively unaffected.

As retinopathy can become quite advanced before it notably affects the sight, it is essential that everyone with diabetes has regular screening for retinopathy. This entails having a photograph taken of the back of the eyes, usually once a year, using a camera that looks through the pupil. Screening is often provided by high street optometrists or by mobile units that run screening sessions at different locations. It is free of charge. The good news is that if retinopathy is picked up early, then treatment is available to stop it progressing to the stage where it can affect vision. Laser therapy is the traditional form of treatment: a fine laser beam is shone through the pupil to the areas of retina affected and works by stopping the damaged retina producing the chemical signals that lead to the formation of new blood vessels. It can also help shrink any blood vessels that have already formed and is very effective in preventing blindness.

Recently, newer treatments have become available to treat maculopathy. These are given by injection through the front of the eye into the macula, and are a class of drugs known as anti-VEGF (vascular endothelial growth factor); they can be very effective in protecting vision, particularly when the macula is swollen (macular oedema).

The other piece of good news is that retinopathy can be prevented by maintaining good control of diabetes and blood pressure, and by stopping smoking. While very mild background retinopathy is not that uncommon in people with longstanding diabetes, sight-threatening retinopathy is almost unheard of in people whose diabetes is well controlled. Further useful information on retinopathy is available at the UK retinopathy screening service website.[1]

DIABETIC KIDNEY DISEASE – NEPHROPATHY

The other part of the body that is particularly affected by small vessel disease is the kidney. The kidneys are the essential organs that help maintain the correct balance of chemicals, salts and water in the bloodstream. As the heart pumps blood around the body it passes through the kidneys that sit on either side of the back, just below the ribs. Whereas in most tissues capillaries transfer nutrients to the surrounding cells, the reverse occurs in the kidneys. Here, specialised capillaries transfer waste products into tiny tubes called collecting ducts. These then lead into the ureter, which takes the waste (urine) into the bladder.

Let's take glucose as an example: when the level of glucose in the bloodstream rises above about 10mmol/l the kidneys try to get rid of the excess glucose by removing it into the urine. This glucose has to be dissolved in water so the kidneys release extra water into the urine. This naturally results in making the individual pass more urine, leading to dehydration, which in turn causes an obvious thirst and an urge to drink more fluid in an attempt to keep well hydrated. So the common symptoms of high glucose levels, namely excess thirst and urination, are the result of the kidneys doing their job in trying to restore more normal levels of glucose in the blood.

The kidneys act like a filter or a fine sieve, allowing only certain things through and into the urine. When the capillaries in the kidney become damaged, the filter becomes leaky (or the holes in the sieve become larger) and this allows substances (such as proteins), which normally should be kept in the bloodstream, to leak out into the urine. So finding the presence of protein in the urine can be a sign that the kidneys have been affected by diabetes.

Just leaking a little extra protein in the urine is in itself of little consequence. However, over time, diabetic kidney disease can cause the pressure within the kidneys to rise, which can increase their leakiness. Kidneys are also important in controlling blood pressure, and damage to them can cause the blood pressure to rise, which in turn can increase the pressure in the kidneys, so causing additional damage. Eventually the kidneys can become seriously damaged and even scarred, making them ineffective in maintaining the correct composition of the blood. This eventually leads to kidney failure and the need for dialysis or a kidney transplant.

Fortunately, just as with diabetic eye disease, this severe form of kidney disease is increasingly rare, and with good care, kidney disease can be prevented. The message is the same and worth repeating: keeping good control of diabetes and blood pressure will avoid these problems. It is important to have a urine test once a year to check if there is any sign of protein leaking into the urine, and if there is, treatments are now available which can help reverse this leak and keep the kidneys healthy. Even people whose kidney function has been moderately affected by diabetes can lead long and active lives thanks to treatments that control blood pressure and prevent any further damage. The commonest type of such treatment is a class of drugs called ACE inhibitors (such as ramipril or lisinopril for example). They work by reducing the pressure within the kidneys and as a result can reduce the leak of protein into the urine, helping maintain good kidney function.

DIABETIC NEUROPATHY – NERVE DISEASE

If the blood vessels are a bit like the heating system in your house, the nerves are analogous to the electrical wiring, providing information (sensation) from all parts of the body and power to all the muscles of the body. In fact, nerves are specialised cells whose function is to transmit tiny electrical currents from one end to the other, so they do act a bit like electrical wires.

So-called sensory nerves have specialised endings in the tissues that pick up a particular sensation. If, for example, you step on a sharp object such as a pin, nerve endings in the skin will transmit the pain sensation up your leg, up and along the spinal cord to the brain. While the pain itself is unpleasant, it is in fact acting as a protective mechanism for your foot. Within the brain nerves will connect to the area that controls speech, so that you may well shout 'ouch' or something rather less polite. They will also connect to motor nerves that travel back down the spinal cord, and to the muscles in your leg that now contract quickly to lift your foot away from the painful object. Sensory and motor nerves control just about every function in the body, from the beating of the heart, to the movement of the gut, sweating, sexual function, emptying the bladder and just about everything else.

In diabetes nerve function can be affected by high glucose levels, both in the short and long term. The short-term effects can be likened to a toxic effect of glucose on the nerves and it is not unusual for people to describe a tingling in the feet, or the difficulty of getting an erection during periods when their glucose levels are high – and for these symptoms to improve once the glucose levels stabilise. In the longer term more permanent nerve damage can occur as a result of high glucose levels. There are a number of possible mechanisms for this and it is likely that the accumulation of glucose within the nerves causes direct damage, as well as nerves being affected by damage to the small blood vessels that supply them.

The longest nerves tend to be affected first and in most people these are the nerves to the feet followed by those to the hands. As a result the most well-known type of neuropathy is that which affects the sensory nerves in the feet. This can lead to tingling and gradually to loss of sensation, so that the feet become essentially numb. The risk here is that stepping on a sharp object won't be registered as pain, and this, in turn, may lead to the injury being left untended. Infection may then set in and might lead to ulceration and more extensive damage to the whole foot. If there is also large vessel disease affecting the circulation, then such injuries can be very difficult to heal, and it is this combination that can, in some cases, lead to a need for amputation.

While loss of sensation is perhaps the most common nerve problem in diabetes, the opposite can also occur, where the nerve endings become over-stimulated to cause unpleasant tingling or painful sensations. In some cases, these can be improved by good glucose control, but often sufferers need to take medication to reduce the unpleasant sensations (see table on p. 43).

There are no treatments that can delay or reverse nerve damage and so, as with other types of complication, the key is to prevent it in the first place – by maintaining good control of blood glucose levels. It is important to have your feet examined at least once a year, and more frequently if there is any sign of nerve damage. Hopefully there will never be any problems, but at the first sign of any sensory problems, it is vitally important to take very great care of your feet in order to minimise any more extensive damage.

Since nerves supply every part of the body, many different body functions can be affected by diabetic nerve damage. One of the most common is for men to find it difficult to get an erection. Treatments such as Viagra can be very helpful. More extensive disease can affect the sweat glands, causing excessive sweating; the bladder causing frequent urination or difficulty in passing water; and the gut to cause problems such as heartburn, diarrhoea or constipation. Specific treatments are available which can be helpful for these problems, as shown in the table opposite.

Discussion about the long-term complications of diabetes is not easy as, to be frank, they are not very pleasant. However, I do believe it is essential that everyone with diabetes knows about them, as appropriate lifestyle changes early on can greatly help achieve good control of glucose levels and that is the key to preventing them ever

DRUGS USED TO TREAT SYMPTOMS OF NEUROPATHY

Symptom	Cause	Treatments available
Erectile dysfunction	Damage to nerves to penis	Sildenafil (Viagra), tadalafil (Cialis), vardenafil (Levitra), Caverject injections
Excessive sweating	Damage to nerves to sweat glands	Oxybutynin
Heartburn	Reflux of acid into oesophagus	Antacids Omeprazole, lansoprazole
Regurgitation of food	Stomach not emptying properly	Domperidone, metoclopramide
Diarrhoea	Disordered gut motility, overgrowth of bacteria in gut	Codeine phosphate Short course of antibiotic (e.g. tetracycline)
Constipation	Loss of sensation in lower bowel	Standard laxatives, e.g. lactulose, senna
Painful symptoms e.g. shooting pains, pins and needles	Hypersensitivity of nerves carrying pain sensation	Duloxetine, amitriptyline, pregabalin, gabapentin
Frequent urination	Bladder irritability	A number of preparations including oxybutynin, solifenacin, tolterodine
Difficulty passing urine	Loss of bladder sensation	Bethanechol chloride; catheterisation
Fainting, light-headedness	Low blood pressure	Fludrocortisone

occurring in the first place. It is also essential that people with diabetes have the regular check-ups that are designed to detect the earliest signs of any of these problems so that they can be treated and, in some cases, even reversed. This will be discussed in more detail in chapter 17. But above all it is important to set these complications into context, to be aware that great advances have been made in our ability to prevent them and to treat them, and that with appropriate support it is perfectly possible to live a long and happy life with diabetes without the emergence of significant complications.

CHAPTER 4

CONVENTIONAL TREATMENT: DIET, LIFESTYLE AND DRUGS

The traditional approach to the management of type 2 diabetes initially focused on changes to diet. The aim was to enable people to lose weight and at the same time to stabilise their blood glucose levels. In the early days diabetes was seen as a problem with glucose, and the promoted diet, therefore, focused on restricting carbohydrates (i.e. foods containing sugars or starches) as these are converted into glucose in the gut. However, by the 1970s doctors were concerned that a diet that was low in carbohydrates was necessarily high in fat. And by then the tide was turning against fat: it was seen as causing high cholesterol levels, heart disease and obesity.

A healthy diet was considered to be one that was low in fat and high in carbohydrates, and it was a natural evolution that the medical community came to believe that people with type 2 diabetes should follow a healthy diet, rather than focus on reducing carbohydrates.

As well as fat being considered unhealthy it was felt that protein might also be problematic. Protein is broken down in the body into creatinine, and will accumulate in patients with kidney failure. As some people with diabetes can have kidney problems, it was felt a high-protein diet ought to be avoided, and this further led to the focus on carbohydrates as the main source of energy.

There was also little distinction between type 1 and type 2 diabetes and it was only in the 1970s that evidence began to emerge that they were separate conditions. People with type 1 diabetes were treated with insulin, usually with one or two injections a day, and in order to avoid their glucose levels falling too low, it was recommended that they eat snacks between each meal and to eat carbohydrates with every meal. This thinking also influenced the recommended diet for people with type 2 diabetes, which by the early 1980s was as follows:

- eat small frequent meals
- eat carbohydrates with each meal
- carbohydrates should form at least 50 per cent of all energy (calories) consumed
- complex carbohydrates (e.g. starches) should be eaten rather than simple carbohydrates such as sugars

- the diet should be high in fibre and low in fat
- calorie intake should be restricted to enable people to lose weight

The result has been that anyone diagnosed with diabetes in the past 30 years will have been advised to follow this type of diet, and until recently this was still the official recommendation found in publications and on websites from organisations such as Diabetes UK.

However, there has been very little information available of a consistently high standard that informs people about what this diet actually means in practice. Many diagnosed with the condition would not have access to a dietitian, and patient education was either haphazard at best, or non-existent at worst. As a result, it was perfectly possible that people made very few changes to their diet, and may even have increased their carbohydrate intake, if previously they had not eaten carbohydrates with every meal.

At the same time as following this diet patients were encouraged to increase their physical activity levels, and 'diet and exercise' were often mentioned together as the initial treatment for type 2 diabetes. Again very little quality information was provided about what this would mean in practice, and unless patients were especially motivated (and curious enough to conduct their own research) to make lifestyle changes, many simply carried on as before.

It is probably not so surprising then that 'diet and exercise' were often ineffective in controlling blood glucose levels, and when the inevitable loss of control arose, medication was needed. Until the 1950s this meant taking insulin injections, but subsequently a class of drugs was discovered that helps the pancreas produce more insulin.

SULFONYLUREAS

Sulfonylureas are a group of drugs that stimulate the pancreas to produce more insulin. They were discovered by accident during research into the effects of antibiotics called sulphonamides that were being developed as a treatment for typhoid fever during the Second World War. A number of patients developed side effects that later were discovered to be linked to low blood glucose levels. The first sulfonylurea to be developed was tolbutamide, released in 1956, and since then a number of different sulfonylureas have been produced; those currently used are listed in the table below.

Sulfonylureas soon became accepted as an effective alternative to insulin injections and were widely prescribed by the end of the 20th century. They were generally well tolerated with few side effects, and were found to be effective in reducing blood glucose levels in people whose diabetes could not be controlled by following the recommended diet.

SULPHONYLUREAS IN USE IN 2014

Name	Dose – taken with meals	Notes
Glibenclamide	2.5–20mg once a day	Very long acting, not suitable for elderly patients
Glipizide	2.5–10mg once or twice a day	
Gliclazide	40–160mg once or twice a day	
Glimepiride	1–6mg once a day	
Tolbutamide	250mg–500mg, one to three times a day	Short-acting, suitable for the elderly or those who are physically active

In each case sulfonylureas are generally prescribed at a low dose to start with and then gradually increased as required in order to adequately control glucose levels. It is important to be aware that if the dose is too high sulfonylureas can make the glucose level fall too low (hypoglycaemia). This can occur if a person is prescribed the wrong dose, if they have eaten a meal with less carbohydrate than usual, or if they are physically more active. Such hypoglycaemia can be a particular problem in elderly people whose appetite may reduce over time, or in those with reduced kidney function.

While sulfonylureas are often effective for many years, over time this effect diminishes. It is as though the pancreas becomes exhausted and runs out of insulin, whereupon additional treatment is required. As sulfonylureas increase insulin secretion they do not help the underlying problem of insulin resistance; in fact they may make things worse by causing people to gain weight, and as we shall see in chapter 5, this in itself makes it more difficult to control diabetes.

METFORMIN

Metformin was first introduced in the early 1960s. It is based on a drug that was initially developed as a treatment for malaria; again it was found to reduce glucose levels in the blood. For many years metformin was considered to be of limited use, but was often added to sulfonylureas when they no longer controlled glucose levels. It is not entirely clear how metformin works, but its main effect appears to be to reduce the amount of glucose released from the liver. Unlike sulfonylureas, metformin does not increase the amount of insulin produced – rather it helps make better use of the body's own insulin. In normal circumstances therefore, it does not cause blood glucose levels to fall too low, and as insulin levels are not increased, metformin does not cause people to gain weight. In fact, some people report that it makes them feel less hungry and can therefore help with weight loss. For this reason metformin has become the treatment of choice for people who are overweight (which accounts for the majority of people now diagnosed with type 2 diabetes) and over time it has become apparent that metformin is actually much more effective than was originally thought. It is also extremely safe and has been shown to reduce the risk of heart disease in people with diabetes.

However, metformin can be associated with side effects, most commonly affecting the gut. It is not unusual for people to experience symptoms such as diarrhoea, wind or bloating when they first take metformin. These generally settle once the body has got used to the drug and for this reason it is suggested that people start at a low dose such as 500mg (one tablet) once a day and gradually build up over a period of a few weeks to the maximum dose of 1000mg (two tablets) twice daily. The side effects can be reduced by taking it with meals. Some people find that they can only tolerate a dose of one or two tablets a day. The general advice is to find the dose that you can take without causing troublesome side effects and to stay on that dose – any dose is better than none. There are also slow-release preparations of metformin available that can be taken just once a day. These are said to be kinder on the gut, and many people who cannot tolerate standard metformin, have no problem with slow-release tablets.

However, some people just cannot tolerate any dose of metformin. I have seen people struggle with quite extreme side effects including abdominal pain and chronic diarrhoea, and some who have even had a colonoscopy (an examination of the large bowel performed by passing an endoscope through the anus) before someone has realised metformin may be the culprit. I always advise that if troublesome side effects persist, metformin should be stopped and another way found to treat the diabetes. Diabetes treatment is meant to make life better – not worse.

Another potential problem with metformin is a rare condition called lactic acidosis. This is where lactic acid builds up in the bloodstream. This usually occurs in people with kidney, heart or liver problems, or with serious infections. It has been observed that lactic acidosis can be more severe in patients who take metformin, and for this reason metformin was often withheld in people who had these medical problems. It has since become apparent that metformin is an extremely safe drug, and is unlikely to be the cause of lactic acidosis, so it is now more commonly prescribed than previously.

The one remaining area of concern is in patients with renal failure, where the risk of lactic acidosis is significant, especially if they become unwell with an infection, for example. For this reason people taking metformin are advised to stop it if they are admitted urgently to hospital or if they should become dehydrated, as a result of diarrhoea and/or vomiting. It can generally be restarted on recovery. There is much confusion about the effect of metformin on kidney function, and in many cases metformin is blamed for kidney problems. This is hardly ever the case. It is just that kidney function needs to be above a certain level (expressed as a blood test called eGFR of at least 30) in order for metformin to be taken safely. Even having said that, for the vast majority of people, metformin is a remarkably safe and effective drug.

In a number of cases, glucose levels remain elevated, despite taking both metformin and one of the sulfonylurea drugs. In these cases until the early 2000s the only option was insulin injections. There are many different types of insulin and a detailed description of insulin is not within the scope of this book. The most common insulin regimens in type 2 diabetes are an injection once or twice daily. Until the 1990s it was common practice to stop tablets and continue just with insulin treatment, but it has since become apparent that continuing metformin means a lower insulin dose is required to achieve good glucose control. In some cases sulfonylureas are also continued with insulin treatment.

HYPOGLYCAEMIA

Hypoglycaemia is the term used to describe an abnormally low blood glucose level, which, for practical purposes means a level below 4mmol/l. Glucose levels rarely fall much lower than this in people without diabetes, but for those who are on medication that actively lowers glucose levels, such as insulin or a sulfonylurea, then it is possible that if the dose is too high, glucose levels can be driven down to dangerously low levels (for example, less than 2mmol/l). The reason why this is so dangerous is that at these low levels the brain cannot function as normal. Hypoglycaemia is associated with two different types of symptoms: the first, which occur when glucose levels are around 3mmol/l, are a result of the body releasing adrenaline and other hormones in an attempt to increase glucose levels and include sweating, shakiness and hunger. When glucose levels fall lower, a second type of symptom occurs that is a result of the brain not receiving enough energy, and includes drowsiness, poor concentration and slurred speech. It is not unusual for these to be mistaken for drunkenness. Extreme hypoglycaemia can lead to fitting and unconsciousness.

Hypoglycaemia is without doubt a very nasty experience, and every effort should be made to ensure it does not happen. Fortunately, most types of treatment for type 2 diabetes do not cause hypoglycaemia. However, both insulin and sulfonylureas will cause hypoglycaemia if the dose taken is too high. It is therefore of the utmost importance that people taking these medications are on the correct dose, that they measure their blood glucose on a regular basis and that they know the symptoms of hypoglycaemia and how to treat it. The recommended treatment is to take 15–20g of fast-acting carbohydrates as shown in the table:

Food	15g carbohydrate is found in:
Glucose/dextrose tablets	5
Lucozade	80ml
Sports drinks e.g. Lucozade Sport	230ml
Cola-type fizzy drink	150ml
Jelly babies	5
Jelly beans	10
Fruit pastilles	6

This should be followed by a longer-acting carbohydrate such as a cheese sandwich.

If you experience hypoglycaemia on a regular basis, or if your glucose levels are often below 4mmol/l, then it is important to ask your diabetes team to review your medication.

When starting out on insulin, people with type 2 diabetes often achieve stable control for a while but then find they need to keep increasing the insulin dose in order to maintain that control. Insulin treatment is also associated with weight gain, and it is not unusual for people to find themselves in a vicious circle of needing to increase the dose of insulin, leading to increased weight, which in turn requires more insulin. Given that the main problem in most cases of type 2 diabetes is insulin resistance, that is the body is unable to use insulin effectively, then taking insulin at ever-increasing doses seems an illogical treatment. For this reason a number of new treatments for type 2 diabetes became available in the 2000s. Some were ineffective and downright dangerous. Others were remarkably effective and began quite fundamentally to change the way we viewed the treatment of type 2 diabetes. These are described in more detail in chapter 14.

CHAPTER 5

THE DIABETES AND OBESITY EPIDEMIC

There is no doubt that the past 10 years has seen a massive increase in the number of people with diabetes, and also in the number of those who are obese. In chapter 2 we described how the diagnosis of diabetes is made on the basis of blood glucose levels. Obesity is diagnosed by calculating an individual's body mass index (BMI). This is the relationship between a person's height and their weight. Normal body weight is defined as a body mass index between 20 and 25. A BMI between 25 and 30 is defined as overweight and above 30 as obese. The precise calculation is to take the weight in kilograms and to divide it by the square of the height in metres. So for a person who weighs 80 kilos (about 12.5 stone) and is 1.83m tall (about 6 feet), the BMI is calculated as:

▶ 80/(1.83x1.83) = 23.9 (which would be in the normal range).

A person of the same height who weighs 110 kilos (about 17 stone) has a BMI of 110/(1.83x1.83) = 32.9, which is in the obese range. A chart to help work out your BMI is in appendix 2.

The BMI is generally not used for children and care must be taken with individuals who are very muscular. Muscle weighs more than fat, and it is quite possible for someone to be 'overweight' but actually very fit and healthy, with an increased body weight because of large muscles. It has been suggested that waist circumference is a better measure of obesity as most people who are genuinely overweight owing to fat have large fat stores around their middle. A few years ago we asked some local general practices to identify people using this definition – and discovered that none of them were recording the data. It is much easier to get someone to stand on scales to measure their weight than pass a tape measure round their middle, and for most purposes BMI is used as a reliable indicator of obesity.

Until the 1990s, type 2 diabetes was not readily associated with obesity. Certainly there were people who were obese and had type 2 diabetes, but there were also many people with type 2 diabetes who, while a little overweight, were not obese at diagnosis.

I know this because in 1993 an education programme for people newly diagnosed with diabetes was implemented in the Bournemouth hospital where I worked. Everybody who was diagnosed by their GP as having diabetes was referred to the diabetes centre within a week of the diagnosis in order to attend three education sessions over the next few weeks. At the first session everyone was weighed and detailed records were kept on all patients with new-onset type 2 diabetes until the programme transferred out of our centre in 2005. In 1995 there were thought to be about one million people in the UK with type 2 diabetes. During that year 367 people newly diagnosed with type 2 diabetes were referred to our education programme. Their average body weight was 82 kilos with a BMI of 29, which is in the overweight range.

What happened over the next 10 years was striking. Firstly there was a steady increase in the number of people diagnosed with type 2 diabetes, so that in the year 2000 nearly 800 people attended the education programme, and by then the total number of cases in the UK had doubled to two million. There had been a slight increase in the average weight of our newly diagnosed patients to 84.5 kilos. For the next few years the numbers with newly diagnosed diabetes in the Bournemouth area remained between 700–800 each year, but their weight continued to increase, and by 2005 the average weight was 89 kilos, over 7 kilos (or a stone) heavier than their counterparts who had been diagnosed 10 years earlier. By then hardly anyone was of normal body weight. Type 2 diabetes had become a disease of the overweight and obese, much like the very early historical accounts of the disease. And by 2013, there were over three million people in the United Kingdom with type 2 diabetes – and it is estimated that over 30 per cent of the population were obese.

This has led to a big shift in the way we think about the disease. In the 1990s people were reassured that they did not get diabetes as a result of their diet or lifestyle. Rather, their diabetes was due to unknown factors and beyond their control, perhaps in their genes. However (perversely), they were also told changing their lifestyle would help control it. Twenty years later, with the twin epidemics of diabetes and obesity visited upon us, and the close correlation between the two, it is abundantly clear that in many cases diabetes has developed in individuals as a result of them being overweight. And for the number of people developing diabetes to have increased so much in just a few years means it cannot be due to some sort of genetic disposition alone. The message is now very clear: if you eat too much and/or exercise too little, you will become overweight. And if you become overweight there is a greatly increased chance of developing diabetes. The bad news is that on an individual level this means there is a direct link between a person's lifestyle and later development of diabetes; the good news is that this readily explains why lifestyle changes can help control diabetes – and raises the possibility that changing lifestyle might help reverse the condition.

Let me just add that while the majority of people with type 2 diabetes are overweight, I would reiterate the points made in chapter 2: some people are not overweight when they develop diabetes. In some cases, these may represent people with a different form of the disease, and may require insulin at some point to control their diabetes. Alternatively they could have excess fat in the abdomen, the significance of this is described later in this chapter, yet still have a normal body weight. There is also interesting evidence which suggests that consuming excess sugar may contribute to the development of diabetes, even in people who are not overweight. This will be discussed further in chapter 9.

We should not be surprised that the increase in obesity in the UK has been associated with an increase in type 2 diabetes as similar stories have been reported in different parts of the world, where lifestyle changes have led to big increases in the prevalence of diabetes. One of the most well-known cases is that of the Pima Indians who live in Arizona in the United States.

Until the early 1900s Pima Indians lived on a predominantly vegetarian low-fat diet derived from crops grown in irrigated areas of the Arizona desert. With the coming of white farmers, water was diverted from the Pima irrigation systems, resulting in crop failures and starvation. The Pima Indians became dependent on a Western diet that is high in fat and refined carbohydrates. This, together with the reduced physical activity resulting from the loss of farming, led to rapid increases in obesity among the Pima population and has now reached epidemic proportions, with over 90 per cent being obese, and over 50 per cent having type 2 diabetes. Interestingly, there is a related population of Pima Indians in Mexico who still follow a traditional lifestyle and diet and who have much lower rates of obesity and diabetes.[1]

Now, while it appears that Pima Indians have a genetic tendency to develop type 2 diabetes, it is clear that diabetes only developed in the presence of obesity. A possible explanation for this is the so-called 'thrifty genotype' hypothesis. This states that populations that rely on traditional sources of food (so-called hunter-gatherers) are readily able to store fat during times when food is abundant. They can then make use of these fat stores when food is scarce. This is a great asset in a traditional setting; however, in an industrialised society, where high-calorie food is readily available, the excess calories are still stored as fat. There are rarely, if ever, periods of famine when these stores will be used up, and so fat continues to accumulate – leading to obesity. This is exacerbated by the lack of physical activity (so fewer calories are burned off) that characterises Western society and other urban societies.

This problem is not confined to Pima Indians. Many thousands of miles away in the South Pacific lies the Micronesian island of Nauru that is a mere 8.5 square miles. For thousands of years its small indigenous population lived off fish, meat and local fruits and vegetables, and were said by early European settlers to be strong, muscular and mostly in good health.

This continued until the Second World War when the Japanese invaded the island. This led to a period during which indigenous agriculture was abandoned and the population became dependent on imported, mostly Western, foods. As with the Pima Indians this led to a high prevalence of obesity and type 2 diabetes.[2]

While the traditional diets of the Pima and Nauru populations were in detail quite different, the overriding similarity was that they were both relatively low in fat and refined carbohydrates and, most importantly, low in calories.

THE 21ST-CENTURY PLAGUE

What we are now seeing is that this epidemic of diabetes seen in faraway places is occurring not only in the UK and other Western countries, but also in many African and Asian countries, where more and more people live in cities and eat high-calorie foods. As we learned in chapter 2, diabetes was considered a rare disease and until the 1950s, occurring in less than 1 per cent of people in almost all countries of the world. In the UK this has now jumped to over 6 per cent and in the USA to nearly 11 per cent, according to the most recent International Diabetes Federation Atlas, which estimates that 8 per cent of the world's population now has diabetes.[3] In 2010, David R Matthews, Professor of Diabetic Medicine at the University of Oxford, gave a lecture during which he drew a forceful comparison between the rise in type

2 diabetes and the medieval pandemic known as the Black Death (likely to have been bubonic plague caused by a bacterium called *Yersinia pestis* that is carried by fleas) and the spread of which was facilitated by the contemporary living environment of overcrowding and poor sanitation.[4] The plague swept across Europe in the 14th century peaking between 1348–50, and resulting in tens of millions of deaths. In the case of obesity and type 2 diabetes the cause (or vector) is calorie excess (that is eating too much), spread by the availability of high-calorie foods at low cost in the context of a changed environment which encourages an unhealthy, sedentary lifestyle. The rapid rise in obesity and diabetes cannot be due to changes in our genes, and so we have to accept that it is due to changes in diet and lifestyle. The tragedy is that if left unchecked, this modern epidemic will prove every bit as catastrophic as the original plague.

So simply put, we are gaining weight because of calories. Or more specifically the balance between the calories we eat and drink and the calories we use up by being active – or do not use up by being insufficiently active. Although, if you have diabetes, your eating habits are likely to have played a role, it would not be right to blame yourself entirely for having developed diabetes. It is important to remember that this is a problem affecting millions of people across the world, which has come about as a result of the advances in agriculture and the overall increase in wealth that have affected, and in many ways benefitted, us all. Technology, scientific and social advances mean the world's growing population has access to more high-calorie food to eat. Those same technological advances mean that our physical activity levels are much lower than those of our predecessors. Stop and have a think about your current levels of activity, and those of your childhood, or perhaps of your parents when they were your age. There are obvious differences, such as the increased use of the car (two-car families were quite unusual when I was a child in the 1960s; if one parent was out at work, the other had to walk the children to and from school). Housewives bought food from a number of different shops and sometimes bought it fresh every day. This often required quite a lot of walking, rather than a weekly drive to the supermarket. There has also been a significant decline in physically demanding industrial jobs, many of which have been replaced by jobs that involve sitting at a computer all day.

Then there are more subtle differences such as the use of the television remote control that means you have a whole array of entertainment at your fingertips (in the old days you had to get up and walk to the television to switch channels); the use of escalators and lifts (in some hotels it is almost impossible to find the stairs); the use of computers, which means that children no longer need to go outside for entertainment and adventure and adults can stay at home and do all their shopping, banking and even socialising online.

And at the same time that all this has been happening, food has become ever more plentiful and cheaper. At a time of rising prices and austerity it may be difficult to remember that in the 1970s food was in real terms more expensive than it is now. Crisps and fizzy drinks (both high in calories) used to be a treat for children, whereas now they form part of many people's everyday lunch. In fact a packet of crisps is now cheaper in major supermarkets than a single apple. Eating out used to be an expensive occasional event. Fast food hadn't been invented – I remember eating in the very first McDonald's in London in the late 1970s. A friend of mine said they would never last as there were no knives and forks! And snack-type food is now available everywhere; whenever I travel to London by train, and arrive at a main station I have to resist the temptations of several outlets selling all manner of high-calorie foods, whereas in the 1970s there was one rather uninspiring cafeteria.

It is the same story on our high streets, where fast-food chains and coffee shops are in abundance. Even some hospitals have fast-food outlets inside them. Thinking about these changes isn't just a case of nostalgia, but rather it should help you see how our modern environment has changed so dramatically since the hunger that was prevalent up until the Second World War, and how, without much in the way of countering forces, it has inadvertently but inevitably encouraged the spread of obesity. Understanding this brief but important history of cultural shift can be used to identify whether we can, individually, undo some of the consequences of the more damaging changes in order to begin to live more healthy lives. We will cover this is more detail in chapters 7 to 9.

The changes to diet and activity levels have also led to a big increase in rates of obesity in young children in the UK. By 2010, nearly one in four (23.1 per cent) of all four- to five-year-olds were classified as overweight or obese, and this trend increases steadily through the primary school years, to 1 in 3 (33.4 per cent) by the age of 10 to 11. As a result we are already seeing cases of type 2 diabetes in children and young adults; this represents a dramatic evolution from a condition that used to be considered as one affecting those over 40 years of age. It also raises the alarming prospect that, for the first time in living memory, the current generation of children may have a poorer health and life-expectancy outlook than their parents.

In summary, then, there is clear evidence that as a result of changes in lifestyle from a young age people are taking in more calories than they are using up (more food and less activity), and as a result they are putting on weight. Carrying excess weight leads to insulin resistance and this is what eventually leads to diabetes (as described in chapter 2). However, quite how that happens has always remained something of a mystery.

FAT IN THE LIVER

If we consume more than we need then the human body is very efficient at storing the excess energy as fat. We all know that if we put on weight we become a bit chubbier due to increased fat tissue below the skin. This is what causes a double chin, for example. We also know that men in particular are prone to carry fat around the middle, the so-called beer belly. This fat is in the abdominal cavity and surrounds organs such as the gut. With the advent of body scanning it has become apparent that many people who are overweight develop what is termed fatty liver, which is just that – excess fat deposited in the liver itself. We have known for some time that people with fatty liver may show evidence that their liver function is affected, not in a dangerous way, but enough to show up on blood tests of so-called liver enzymes, such as alanine aminotransferase (ALT) or aspartate transaminase (AST), whose levels are raised. Occasionally, fatty liver can progress to cirrhosis, which is associated with permanent scarring of, and damage to, the liver.

Research published in 2011 by Professor Roy Taylor of Newcastle University[5] suggested that this excess fat in the liver is very significant in the development of diabetes. His work suggests there is a vicious circle, whereby the excess fat in the liver makes the liver resistant to insulin. This means that insulin can no longer stop glucose leaving the liver and entering the bloodstream (the insulin 'tap' becomes leaky letting glucose levels rise in the blood). In order to compensate for this the pancreas produces more insulin. However, one of the effects of high insulin levels is that even more fat is then deposited in the liver, which in turn makes the problem even worse. Over time not only does the liver become filled with fat, but so does the pancreas. And just as a liver full of fat cannot work properly, a pancreas, which is filled with fat, can no longer produce insulin. Although this may not explain every case of type 2 diabetes, the theory does explains how, in many people, obesity leads to diabetes – first by making the liver resistant to insulin, so that blood glucose levels rise, and then by affecting the pancreas so that it cannot produce any more insulin.

CHAPTER 6

CAN DIABETES BE REVERSED?

In the previous chapter we learned how the rapid increase in diabetes is due to the increase in obesity in different populations around the world. This raises an intriguing question: if a person develops diabetes after they become overweight, will they still have diabetes if they lose weight?

In chapter 2 I described how diabetes is diagnosed on the basis of blood tests and that there exists a pre-diabetic condition called impaired glucose tolerance or IGT. In the 1990s it was assumed that people with impaired glucose tolerance would inevitably develop diabetes and there was not much that could be done to stop it. If people with IGT turned up at our education programme for newly diagnosed diabetes we would send them home and tell them to come back when they had developed full-blown diabetes. I imagine that can't have made them feel too good, but that was the medical fraternity's belief at the time.

Things began to change with the emergence of evidence from a number of studies in the early 2000s that demonstrated diabetes could be prevented. The first study was the Diabetes Prevention Program, in the United States, which was published in 2002 in the *New England Journal of Medicine*.[1] In this study, people with IGT were randomly split into different treatment groups. The first group, called the lifestyle intervention group, received advice from an individual case manager for 16 weeks on how to change their diet and lifestyle with the aim of losing weight. They were specifically advised to follow a low-fat, low-calorie diet and to exercise for 30 minutes at least five times a week. The second group received the drug metformin (discussed in chapter 4) and the third group – the control group – received a dummy (placebo) pill. All participants were followed up for four years, during which those in the lifestyle intervention group were reviewed every month to check on their progress. The results were striking: in each year of the study, 5 per cent of the lifestyle intervention group developed diabetes compared to 11 per cent in the placebo group. Those taking metformin were somewhere between the two. The researchers then went back to check up on the participants 10 years after the beginning of the study, and although the intervention had stopped after four years, the benefits continued with a 43 per cent reduction in diabetes in the lifestyle intervention group compared to the control group.

The other main prevention trial was the Finnish Diabetes Prevention Study, published in 2003.[2] This provided similar advice but less intensively (seven sessions in the first year and then every three months for three years), with exercise sessions provided free of charge to participants. Over three years, 9 per cent of subjects developed diabetes compared to 20 per cent in a control group (who did not receive the same advice). In other words, the risk of developing diabetes was reduced by over 50 per cent. The very strong message from these studies is that diabetes can be prevented by losing weight, and that diet and exercise are more effective than medication.

So impressed were we with these data that we set up a pilot study in Bournemouth. People with impaired glucose tolerance were identified at a GP's surgery and they attended a programme of four sessions on diet and exercise, followed by monthly review groups. Not only did these patients then not progress to diabetes, after one year their glucose tolerance test had returned to normal. While we were very encouraged by these results, we were rather discouraged that the local Primary Care Trust, who determine what services should be provided in their area, did not feel setting up such a programme was important enough. The fact remains, however, that this showed that not only could diabetes be prevented, but impaired glucose tolerance could be reversed.

The rise in obesity (as well as type 2 diabetes) is also affecting young children, and, as we learnt in chapter 5, rates of overweight and obese children increase through the primary school years. In 2002 a project was undertaken in local schools to teach children about the risks of drinking sweetened carbonated drinks. The intervention group received the teaching (four lessons over one year) and a control group did not. Over the following year the number of children in the control group who were shown to be overweight or obese increased; there was no such increase in the intervention group.[3] This again suggests that changing behaviour (in this case, children drinking fewer sweetened drinks) can reduce the risk of obesity, and by implication, type 2 diabetes.

The progression from 'normal' through 'impaired glucose tolerance' to 'diabetes' is a continual gradual process, with the definitions of each being arbitrarily set. It is not an on–off situation, like, for example, classical type 1 diabetes or lung cancer – where you either have it or you don't. The interventions described above have shown that it is possible to slow down the progression from IGT to diabetes and to reverse it from IGT to normal. The big question is: can the situation be reversed once a person already has diabetes?

Before looking at recent research in the United Kingdom, I would like to go abroad again – this time to Cuba. Cuba is a large island in the Caribbean and home to a population of 11 million people. Until the late 20th century it was also one of the world's largest producers of sugar and with Cubans exhibiting some of the highest sugar consumption in the world. Under Fidel Castro Cuba became a communist society and a comprehensive public health service was developed that resulted in significant benefits to the island's population that saw infant mortality rates tumble and adult life-expectancy increase (both are now better than in the USA). Meanwhile, the more adverse effects of communism led to inefficiencies in industrial production, including the sugar industry, and food shortages. As a result Cuba had to import a number of foodstuffs and many staple foods were rationed. Cuba became heavily dependent on the former Soviet Union for support for its ailing economy.

This support disappeared rapidly after the collapse of the Soviet Union; its disappearance had a catastrophic effect on the Cuban economy resulting in shortages of both food and oil. By 1993 the food shortages meant 27 per cent of Cubans had lost more than 10 per cent of their body weight and the prevalence of obesity halved from 11.9 per cent to 5.4 per cent.[4] The lack of oil meant buses no longer ran and people had to walk or cycle: in fact, more than a million bicycles were distributed to Cubans between 1991 and 1995. The rationing system protected the population from starvation, although vitamin deficiencies ultimately led to neuropathy – nerve damage – in over 50,000 people.

This enforced change in diet and lifestyle led to a significant decline in deaths related to type 2 diabetes (by over 50 per cent) between 1995 and 2002. There was also a 35 per cent reduction in deaths due to heart disease. While it cannot be proved that actual cases of diabetes reversed (this would have required a widespread blood testing programme – not a priority during an economic crisis) the reduction in deaths demonstrates that the weight loss and increased exercise had a beneficial effect on the health of very many people. And as we will see later in this chapter, it is highly likely that in many cases diabetes was reversed.

The economic situation has since improved and with it greater availability of motorised transport and food. By 2010 nearly all the improvements in health had disappeared with 19 per cent of Cubans obese and a near doubling in new cases of diabetes. It is of note that the rationing system is still in place with strict limits on the amount of eggs, meat and milk available to most Cubans.

Item	Ration per person per month
Rice	2.7kg
Beans	570g
White sugar	1.4kg
Dark sugar	1.4kg
Milk	1 litre / day (aged 7 or below)
Eggs	12 (Sept to Dec only)
Beef	500g
Chicken	500g

Source: Wikipedia

However, the allowances for sugar and rice are relatively high, and this explains why the Cuban diet derives around 70 per cent of all calories from carbohydrates.

Historically, diabetes was considered to be irreversible and, once diagnosed, a disease for life. However, over the past 20 years it has become apparent that many people with diabetes who have had bariatric (weight-loss) surgery subsequently lose their diabetes.

Bariatric surgery describes a number of operations that all have the same goal: limiting the amount of calories absorbed through the gut into the bloodstream. There are three common types of surgery undertaken in the UK: laparoscopic (keyhole) adjustable gastric banding, laparoscopic gastric bypass and laparoscopic sleeve gastrectomy.

A gastric bypass is an operation to make the stomach smaller and to shorten the length of small intestine that food passes through. This allows food to bypass most of the stomach and part of the small intestine. This means that a person will only be able to eat small amounts and some of the food won't be fully digested.

A gastric band is an inflatable ring that is placed around the upper part of the stomach. It comprises a circular balloon similar to a tiny tube, which is inflated through a port placed just under the skin. It is adjustable, so can be altered once in place. It can also be taken out if needed. Once in place, the band creates a small pouch from the upper part of the stomach that can only hold a small amount of food, which means that a person eats

Reverse your Diabetes

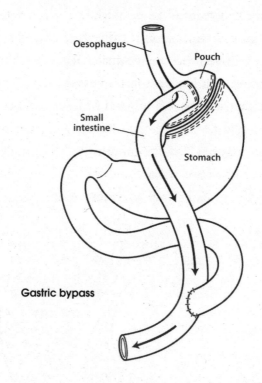

Gastric bypass

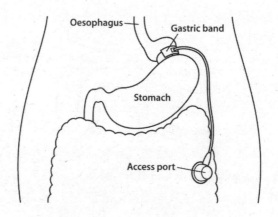

A gastric band

less because they feel full more quickly. The food travels normally through the rest off the digestive system.

The EndoBarrier Gastrointestinal Liner is a relatively new treatment that has demonstrated significant weight loss in clinical trials when combined with certain diet and lifestyle modifications. The EndoBarrier is placed in the gastro intestinal tract via the mouth (endoscopically) to create a barrier between food and the intestine, and to delay the mixing of digestive enzymes with food.

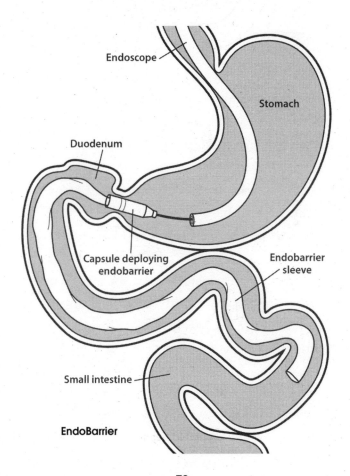

Endoscope

Stomach

Duodenum

Capsule deploying
endobarrier

Endobarrier
sleeve

Small intestine

EndoBarrier

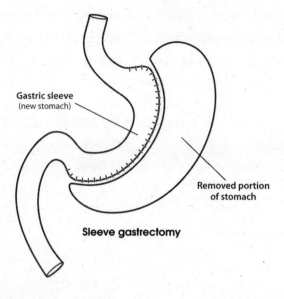

Gastric sleeve
(new stomach)

Removed portion
of stomach

Sleeve gastrectomy

Sleeve gastrectomy is a surgical procedure in which the stomach is reduced to about 25 per cent of its original size by the surgical removal of a large portion of the stomach along the greater curvature, resulting in a sleeve- or tube-like structure. The procedure permanently reduces the size of the stomach and is irreversible.

There have been numerous reports of the effect of such weight-loss procedures on people with diabetes. In one report 72 per cent of people with diabetes had reversed their diabetes by two years, and half of these were still not diabetic after 10 years. There were similar improvements in other aspects of the metabolic syndrome, such as high blood pressure and cholesterol levels. In order to be able to measure the effect of such surgery on reversing diabetes it has become necessary to establish a definition for reversal. In 2009 the American Diabetes Association defined the three stages of diabetes remission: partial, complete or prolonged, depending on the duration and extent of return to normal glucose control without the need for any diabetes medications:

THE THREE STAGES OF DIABETES REVERSAL

	Partial	Complete	Prolonged
Fasting glucose (mmol/l)	<7	<5.6	<5.6
HbA1c (mmol/mol)	<48 (6.5%)	<42 (6.0%)	<42 (6.0%)
Duration (years)	1	1	5

Research from Italy[5] has described the reversal of diabetes in patients who underwent a type of gastric bypass operation. As is common after gut surgery the patients were unable to eat and were fed through a drip for the first six days after their operation (a total of 1800 calories per day). What was significant was that by day seven patients had already lost 6kg in weight and their glucose tolerance test was normal. This weight loss and reversal of diabetes could not have been the result of the operation as it mostly occurred before they had started eating, so they were not even using their new gut. It was more likely their diabetes had reversed as they were unable to eat and instead were on a drip, which did not give them enough calories to maintain their pre-operation body weight. The weight loss would have been accompanied by loss of fat from the liver (which as we learnt in chapter 2 is an important cause of insulin resistance), which in turn would have enabled insulin to work more effectively in reducing the 'leak' of glucose from the liver into the bloodstream, thus reducing their blood glucose levels to reverse their diabetes.

Professor Roy Taylor of Newcastle University, whose work we described in chapter 5, set out to examine the effect of sudden weight loss on both the fat in the liver and on blood glucose levels in 11 people with established type 2 diabetes. He did this by performing various blood tests and MRI scans to look at the liver and the pancreas of the people in the study. They were then asked to follow a strict 600-calorie-per-day liquid diet for eight weeks. What he found was quite remarkable: within a week blood glucose levels returned to normal and this was accompanied by a big reduction in the amount of fat in the liver. Over the next few weeks the fat content in the pancreas also reduced. By eight weeks the pancreas was producing insulin normally and the liver was no longer resistant to the effect of insulin – the leaky tap had a new washer. Taken together these changes meant the people in the study no longer had diabetes.[6] To quote Professor Taylor: 'Our findings were enormously exciting. We had demonstrated that by changing calorie intake we could change fat levels in the liver and pancreas and return insulin sensitivity and insulin production to normal.'

These experiments confirmed his theory that type 2 diabetes is related to the amount of fat in the liver and in the pancreas. What was even more exciting was the discovery that a reduction in calorie intake could reverse the disease process. This is great news because it means that if you have recently been diagnosed with type 2 diabetes then, by reducing your calorie intake and weight, there is a chance that you can become free from diabetes. Many people have dismissed Professor Taylor's work on the basis that he only looked at a small number of people; that they were required to follow a very low-calorie diet that is not sustainable in the longer term and, after the study, some people regained weight and became diabetic again. However, this rather misses the point in that this was an experiment that proved that weight loss, without bariatric surgery, could lead to reversal of diabetes. Very few people would recommend a very low-calorie diet as a long-term solution to type 2 diabetes, but the evidence would suggest that people who can find an effective means of losing weight and keeping it off over the long term will be able to reverse their diabetes.

While some people in the medical and scientific community are sceptical about reversal of diabetes, the initial results of Professor Taylor's work attracted headlines around the world and caught the imagination of many people who went on to try a similar approach themselves. His team subsequently published details of 77 people who contacted them with their experiences about reversing their diabetes. Reversal of diabetes was considered to have occurred in 61 per cent and was more likely to occur in those who lost most weight and/or had shorter duration of diabetes.[7] A formal study in the US[8] also showed that weight loss was associated with reversal of diabetes – in this study the amount of weight lost was much less, and fewer subjects reversed their diabetes – however, the message is the same, it is possible.

The reversibility of type 2 diabetes is being further explored in a new study, funded by Diabetes UK. The aim of this research, called the DIRECT (DIabetes REmission Clinical Trial) study, is to evaluate the potential for diabetes reversal on a larger scale in a general practice setting, and to compare the long-term effects of the new approach with that of the best diabetes care that is currently available. The diet used in the study will last for between 8 and 20 weeks and consist of approximately 800 calories a day made up of four different soups or shakes per day (carefully designed to provide all essential vitamins and minerals) plus plentiful fluids. The study will help determine how many people can achieve remission of diabetes, and for how long.

The fact that diabetes may return in association with later weight gain emphasises that this is not a permanent 'cure' from diabetes, regardless of lifestyle. Nevertheless I firmly believe that there is enough evidence from the studies already performed to encourage us to pursue reversal of diabetes as the goal of treatment of everyone newly diagnosed with type 2 diabetes. Not everyone may achieve complete reversal, but even partial reversal associated with modest weight loss and lower glucose levels will significantly improve the long-term health outlook for many people. The next section of the book will consider how this can be achieved.

CHAPTER 7

THE IMPORTANCE OF LOSING WEIGHT

In the first part of this book we have learned that in most cases of type 2 diabetes weight gain is a predominant cause and that losing weight can lead to reversal of diabetes. I believe this has profound implications for how type 2 diabetes should be managed. The emphasis should be on lifestyle changes with the aim of losing weight while keeping blood glucose levels under control. This requires a set of self-management skills, including:

▶ Knowing how to achieve weight loss
▶ Knowing how to change your diet
▶ Understanding the importance of regular exercise

➧ Knowing how to use blood glucose testing to check your progress

➧ Knowing which medications to use and when, and which to avoid

The next few chapters will cover each of these topics. We will start with weight loss as this is so critical and the other subjects are linked to it.

In chapter 5 we saw how putting weight on leads directly to type 2 diabetes as a result of the build-up of fat in both the liver and the pancreas. As people lose weight the fat in these organs reduces allowing the organs to work more normally again – and leading to reversal of diabetes. The key to reversing diabetes is therefore to lose weight and to adopt a lifestyle that will help keep glucose levels under control and reduce insulin resistance. This will require regular exercise and changes to the diet.

Our body weight is determined by the difference between the energy we take in (in the form of food and drink) and use up (as physical activity or exercise). So in order to lose weight we need to use up more energy (calories) than we take in. That means for most of us eating less and exercising more.

When I speak of exercise I don't just mean 10-kilometre runs or strenuous workouts at the gym. Any increase in activity, such as walking, housework or gardening, is beneficial. However, while exercise itself can contribute to weight loss, the benefits derived from it are located more in improving overall health and fitness, which in turn helps reduce blood pressure and cholesterol levels. Losing a significant amount of weight cannot be achieved by doing more exercise alone, it also requires changes to your diet. For example, while a 30-minute brisk walk has been shown to have very beneficial effects to health, it uses just one calorie per kilogram of body weight for each kilometre walked. At an average pace one would cover 2.5km in half an hour. So for someone who weighs 100kg (just under 16 stone) the walk will use up 250 calories, which equates to a small bar of chocolate or a small portion of beans on toast – hardly a feast. Someone who weighs 90kg (about 14 stone) will use up even less than this. In addition this level of exercise will have only a modest effect of blood glucose levels, which could be completely undone if it is followed by a meal with carbohydrates in it.

So while exercise is important, managing diabetes really does need to involve changes to what you eat, focusing on reducing the total calorie intake to lose weight and help reverse diabetes in the long term, and also reducing the carbohydrate content of the diet to help keep glucose levels down in the short term.

It has been estimated that in order to reverse diabetes a typical person with type 2 diabetes will need to lose about 15kg (two and a half stone) in weight. Let's be honest, that is a lot of weight to lose. While there are several crash diets which may enable someone to lose this amount of weight very quickly, the risk is that unless the person learns to change their eating habits, once they stop the crash diet, they revert to their previous level of eating and pile the weight back on, sometimes to a higher level than before. Not only are crash diets not always effective, they are not sustainable in the long term and may also not be very healthy as they can be associated with some nutritional deficiencies in the long term.

To lose 15kg requires a long-term commitment and in order to keep up the commitment, the diet has to be sustainable. That is it has to be something you can continue for several months in order to lose the required amount of weight. And once you have reached the desired weight it is important that you do not return to your previous levels of eating, as over time this will mean you ending up right back at square one. Rather than revert to old eating habits, once the initial weight loss has been achieved it is equally important thereafter to eat less than you previously did, in order to balance your food intake with your activity level and keep your weight stable. So the initial diet has to be sustainable while you lose weight, but your eating habits have to change FOR EVER!

Now, if you are not significantly overweight, you may well be thinking that this does not apply to you. Indeed, while the big increase in the number of people with type 2 diabetes is a result of more people weighing more, the internal accumulation of fat that does the damage can occur even in people who are not significantly overweight. This was very well illustrated by Dr Michael Mosley in his book, *The Fast Diet: The Secret of Intermittent Fasting: Lose Weight, Stay Healthy, Live Longer*[1] where he described the benefits of intermittent fasting as a means of losing weight.

Dr Mosley was 180cm (5ft 11ins) tall and weighed 85kg (13 stone 3lb), giving him a body mass index (BMI) of 26. He was only about 5kg (or 11lb) overweight, which by today's standards is not that overweight at all. Although he didn't look particularly fat on the outside those extra pounds of fat were highly visible on an MRI scan and were already affecting his metabolism with high levels of both cholesterol and glucose in his blood. At 7.3mmol/l, his fasting glucose meant that he already had diabetes. After three months he had lost almost 8kg (1½ stone) giving him a BMI of 24. His fasting blood glucose had returned to normal at 5mmol/l with good improvements in his cholesterol levels. This was a direct result of loss of internal fat. He also lost fat from around his neck reducing his collar size and his snoring diminished!

So if, like Dr Mosley, you consider yourself thin on the outside, bear in mind that only a few pounds of excess fat on the inside can have very profound consequences for your metabolism and your health.

Change can be very difficult. By and large we do the things that we like doing and if that includes eating more than we should then eating less may well be difficult. In fact, if it were easy then no one would be overweight! Eating less will be particularly difficult if some of the eating is so-called comfort eating. It is well known that certain foods, such as chocolate, can be associated with chemical changes in the brain that lead to a sense of well-being or even pleasure. Many people who are seriously overweight have a past history of depression or adverse life experiences that have led to eating as a source of comfort. If this is the case, then it is very unlikely that you will be able to change your diet significantly until the underlying problems have been addressed. It is well recognised that type 2 diabetes and depression can occur together and part of this association could be due to the effect of depression causing excess eating, which causes diabetes. This particular topic will be covered in more detail in chapter 20.

Apart from psychological factors, which may get in the way of being able to lose weight, a readiness to change is also very important. If you are to have any chance of succeeding then you must really want to lose weight. Otherwise it just will not happen. Hopefully the prospect of feeling better, and possibly of no longer having diabetes, will be enough motivation. But it may not be. If that is the case, then it may be worth thinking long and hard about whether it is the right time for you to attempt to lose weight. It may be better to wait until you do feel motivated, rather than try and then fail, which will leave you even more disconsolate and reduce what residual motivation you do possess even more.

The next few chapters will give you plenty of ideas for losing weight. Whichever you decide to try it is important to set yourself realistic goals. There is no point setting yourself a goal of losing 15kg if you are simply insufficiently motivated to change your diet. But you could set yourself a small achievable goal: to drink water rather than orange juice, for example, or to stop buying chocolate on weekdays. As you consider some of the options it will be worth identifying what is most important for you. To do this you might like to answer the following questions:

- What are your reasons for reading this book?
- What frustrates you most about having diabetes?
- How do you want things to be different?
- How will you know when you have achieved this?
- What is the main thing you would like to change after reading this book?

We will return to your answers to these questions in chapter 21.

CHAPTER 8

WHY WE EAT WHAT WE EAT

These days we are bombarded with a huge variety of often-conflicting recommendations about the foods we should eat and the foods we should avoid coupled with a seemingly endless litany of health scares about dozens of foods and dangerous food processing and manufacturing practices. It all adds up to a very confusing picture. In truth, humans are very versatile creatures, and historically, populations around the world have always adapted to a diet based on what is or was available in their immediate environment and at that moment. Of necessity, the traditional Eskimo diet was high in fish and sea mammals with very little vegetable intake; on the other had, as we saw in chapter 5, the Pima Indians in Mexico ate a diet that was predominantly based on plant foods. The diet of the Australian aborigines was largely based on plants and witchetty grubs, with an occasional feast of kangaroo meat. Agriculture, which produced refined grain products such as flour, in human evolutionary terms, is a relative newcomer; processed foods, including breakfast cereals that many of us grew up on and might consider 'traditional', as well as 'fast foods', are the very new (and damaging) kids on the block.

We certainly did not evolve to eat chicken nuggets. As Dr John Briffa describes in his excellent book *Escape The Diet Trap*,[1] evidence from prehistoric remains suggests that although ancient human diets differed depending on their environment, they all contained meat, and by today's standards were relatively low in carbohydrates and higher in fat and protein. So why, you may wonder, do modern dietary recommendations place so much emphasis on carbohydrates, and how have traditional natural foods, such as meat and eggs, acquired such a bad name?

My interpretation of the evidence is that in general we are better off eating a diet of natural fresh ingredients as opposed to processed foods. As long as we have a varied and balanced diet, our overall calorie intake is appropriate to our needs, and we do not become overweight, then it is probable that the precise make-up of the diet does not really matter. Remember that in Cuba rates of diabetes fell significantly during food shortages even though the diet was high in sugar. However, if we are eating too many calories, then the evidence really does seem to suggest that carbohydrates (sugar and white rice, for example) make the development of diabetes and obesity more likely. So for people who already have diabetes or obesity (or often both) it makes sense to reduce carbohydrates within a diet based on fresh, natural foods, by making some of the changes suggested in the table:

SUGGESTED FOOD CHANGES

Less	More	Notes
Breakfast cereals	Eggs	
Fruit juice / fizzy drinks	Water	
Processed foods	Fresh meat Fresh or tinned fish	Meat should be eaten in moderation Ham, bacon and cheese are processed foods
Salt		
Sugar		
Chocolate, sweets, cakes, biscuits	Fresh fruit (not tropical fruit) Nuts	Bananas and pineapple are high in sugar
Fruit yoghurt	Plain yoghurt	
Rice, pasta, potatoes	Fresh or frozen vegetables	
Bread (wholemeal, dark rye breads are better than white bread)	Salads and soup	
Low-fat foods	Low-sugar foods	

Now note that the left-hand column says 'less', not 'none'. I love chocolate, cakes and bread (my dad was a baker, after all), but I know I need to eat them sparingly, and as a treat (or in the case of chocolate as an occasional therapy!) Also note that eating too much meat (protein and fat) has also been linked with diabetes. It is unlikely that meat itself causes diabetes, but eating too much meat results in eating too many calories, and through the accumulation of fat will contribute to the development of diabetes.

Our ancestors ate meat once or twice a week at most. Today, in the Western world many people eat meat every day, much of it processed rather than fresh. Buying fresh meat will automatically reduce your intake of the salt and sugar found in processed foods and has the added advantage that you will get what it says on the label. The horse meat scandal in the UK has highlighted how little control we, as consumers, have over what we are eating if it has been transported through several countries and pre-processed and packaged before it appears in the shop.

BUTTER OR MARGARINE?

There is a widespread belief that margarine (made from vegetable oils and several additives) is healthier than butter (made from all-natural ingredients). Standard margarine, as opposed to low-fat spread, has the same amount of fat and calories as butter, and will do nothing to help weight loss. It is true that butter has more saturated fat, which is considered less healthy, but I would prefer to see someone, who is successfully losing weight, enjoy a small amount of butter as part of a natural diet, rather than someone who remains obese and uses margarine.

SUGAR OR SWEETENER?

Refined sugar (as opposed to naturally occurring sugar in fruit for example) is very far from being a natural food, but it is arguably more natural than artificial sweeteners. Given the health problems associated with excess sugar, refined sugar use should be kept to an absolute minimum. Ideally you should learn to enjoy unsweetened drinks, but in the real world there are many people who have a sweet tooth, and who use sweeteners. Their advantage is that they do not affect glucose levels and, as they have no calories, will not directly lead to weight gain or promote diabetes. However, there are fears they pose their own health risks, and interesting evidence from research on mice suggests they may, in some way, stimulate appetite, indirectly leading to weight gain. There are therefore two sides to the argument. On balance, I think that sweeteners used in moderation are likely to be a better option than sugar, but using neither is better still! So, gradually reducing the amount of sugar or sweetener you use will retrain your taste buds so that you do not crave sweet foods so often.

Let's now have a look at individual types of foods and how they can contribute to weight gain and their role in promoting and reversing diabetes.

CHAPTER 9

ALL ABOUT CARBOHYDRATES

In the last chapter I explained that if you have type 2 diabetes, it is likely that you could do with losing some weight – even if you are 'thin on the outside'. There are lots of different approaches to losing weight and many of us will have tried many different types of diet. At the end of the day it doesn't really matter what approach you take, but to be successful a diet must have two important qualities: it needs to involve eating fewer calories than you use up, and it has to lead to a permanent change in your eating habits.

If you have diabetes the aim is not only to lose weight but to reduce your glucose levels as well, and in due course to reverse the disease process. So it is important that the types of food you eat help reduce glucose levels. As we read in chapter 2, the foods that most affect glucose levels are carbohydrate – that is, sugars and starchy foods. So for some time now, my advice to people with type 2 diabetes has been to cut down on carbohydrates. To many people this advice is the complete opposite of what they have been taught in the past, and also runs contrary to much of the current 'official' advice still circulating. Why is that?

For many years we have been actively and loudly encouraged to eat less fat. And in its place we have been told to eat plenty of starchy carbohydrates as these are considered to be less fattening and to contain lots of 'goodness'. In the UK, official government nutritional advice – for everyone, not just those with diabetes – is based on these principles, and, as the extract taken from the NHS Choices: Eight tips for health eating web page makes clear, should include starchy carbohydrates in every meal:[1]

'Base your meals on starchy foods. Starchy foods should make up around one third of the foods you eat. Starchy foods include potatoes, cereals, pasta, rice and bread. Choose wholegrain varieties when you can: they contain more fibre, and can make you feel full for longer. Most of us should eat more starchy foods: try to include at least one starchy food with each main meal. Some people think starchy foods are fattening, but gram for gram they contain fewer than half the calories of fat.'

Note the last sentence that a gram of carbohydrate contains fewer than half the calories of a gram of fat. That is certainly true, but does I think miss the crucial point that encouraging a carbohydrate-based diet can mean that the amount of carbohydrate eaten can easily be over twice that of fat, thus cancelling out the benefit of carbohydrates containing fewer calories. Additionally the conventional line, for many years, has been that people with diabetes should follow the same healthy eating principles as anyone else, and that is why the same advice is given to people with diabetes. Now it may be that this advice is right for the general population (although I would argue that it isn't), but many people in the diabetes community are becoming increasingly convinced that this advice is positively wrong for them. And it is easy to understand why. All starchy carbohydrate is broken down in the gut into glucose, and sugars are broken down into glucose and fructose. We'll come back to fructose later, but for now let us consider what happens to that glucose. It is absorbed from the gut into the bloodstream where, in someone with diabetes, it will cause the glucose level to rise. So every slice of bread, every portion of chips, every portion of rice will cause blood glucose levels to rise – before we even consider the effect of sugars in desserts, cakes and biscuits. That is why the traditional dietary advice for people with diabetes so often makes it difficult to achieve its main goal – normal levels of glucose in the blood.

Not only does this type of recommended diet begin to seem quite nonsensical for someone with diabetes, the evidence is piling up that it might actually help *cause* type 2 diabetes. Many people over the years, when first diagnosed with type 2 diabetes, would ask, 'Is it because I have eaten too much sugar?' And for many years, we would say 'No'. What does recent research show us? First, let us examine the evidence that sugar increases the risk of diabetes.

The Nurses' Health Studies are among the largest and longest-running investigations of factors that influence women's health. Started in 1976 and expanded in 1989, the information provided by the 238,000 dedicated nurse-participants in the United States has led to many new insights on health and disease. Every two years the nurses are sent a questionnaire; nurses (unlike doctors) are very good at filling in forms and over 90 per cent return them completed. The questionnaire asks about their health, including whether they have diabetes, asks for the respondent's body weight and details of their diet, including questions about sugar-sweetened soft drinks, fruit juice and diet soft drinks. Over an eight-year period there were 741 new cases of type 2 diabetes.

The researchers looked at the effect of drinking sweetened drinks on body weight and found that the women who increased their consumption from one drink per week to one or more drinks per day gained an average of 8.9kg over eight years. However, those who reduced their intake of sweetened drinks gained only 1.5kg. As you might expect this had a direct bearing on the development of diabetes, and women who drank at least one drink per day had nearly double the risk of developing type 2 diabetes when compared with those who drank less than one sweetened drink a month.[2] A similar association between consumption of sugar-sweetened drinks and diabetes was reported in a European study, published in 2013. It suggested that one can per day increased the risk of type 2 diabetes by 18 per cent.[3]

Further evidence has come from a study looking at the consumption of high fructose corn syrup (HFCS) – a derivative from the production of corn that is mainly found in food and drinks in the Unites States. It is similar to sucrose (common table sugar that is 50 per cent glucose and 50 per cent fructose), but has at least 10 per cent more fructose than sucrose. In the United States it is much cheaper to produce HFCS than normal sugar and consequently is used in many manufactured foods and drinks. It is used less in the United Kingdom and in some other European countries. In countries with a high HFCS usage, the population is exposed to an extra 10–30 per cent fructose. A recent study has shown that in those countries there are about 20 per cent more cases of diabetes than in those who do not use HFCS.[4] One possible explanation is that fructose has very different effects in the body than glucose. Fructose is taken up into the liver and it has been shown that excess fructose leads to more internal body fat being laid down – especially in the liver. Indeed, the damaging effect of fructose on the liver has been compared to the effect of alcohol.[5] And yet fructose is often cited as being natural, healthy and safe!

An international analysis has shown that the amount of sugar consumed in a country appears to contribute strongly to the prevalence of diabetes in that country, even if obesity levels are quite low. This might explain why some countries, such as France, Bangladesh and the Philippines, have high rates of diabetes despite low levels of obesity. These are markedly different countries in terms of population and wealth, and yet the thing they have in common is a high sugar intake. Conversely, New Zealand has a high rate of obesity, yet a relatively low prevalence of diabetes. This intriguing analysis supports that theory that sugar has a direct effect in causing diabetes.[6] And it is easy to see why – because sugar stimulates release of insulin that in turn stimulates the accumulation of fat in the liver and pancreas. This is the same 'fat on the inside' phenomenon that might explain the development of type 2 diabetes in people who are not overweight.

So we have evidence that consuming high levels of sugar, whether in foods or sweetened drinks, increases the risk of diabetes, as does the use of fructose as a sweetener. The next question to ask is whether a high intake of starchy food may contribute to diabetes. Remember that starchy food is said to be good for us and we are all advised to eat plenty of it. However, in 2012 a study was published that really does call into question this advice. It looked at a number of different research studies to see if there was any evidence that white rice, the staple food in many Asian countries, is linked to diabetes. The answer would seem to be yes and that every serving (about 160g cooked rice) per day of white rice increased the risk of diabetes by around 11 per cent.[7]

Up till now carbohydrates have been divided into sugars and starches, and while sugar intake has always been discouraged, we have been encouraged to eat plenty of starches. As starchy food has to be broken down into sugars before it can be absorbed it had been thought that it had a less marked effect on blood glucose values than eating sugars. However, not all starches are the same. Some starches, such as white rice or mashed potato, are broken down and absorbed as glucose very quickly, in fact almost as quickly as sugar itself. Others, such as brown rice or wholemeal bread, are absorbed much more slowly and have a lesser effect on blood glucose. Glycaemic index (GI) is a term used to describe by how much different carbohydrate-containing foods affect the blood glucose level. Glucose has a GI of 100 and so a food that has a GI of 85 (such as white rice) will have 85 per cent of the effect on the blood glucose level as eating sugar. In contrast, the GI of wholemeal bread is only 53. So if a high intake of sugars has an effect on increasing the risk of diabetes, it comes as no surprise that a high intake of white rice will have a similar effect. We will focus more on glycaemic index later in this chapter.

Okay, you might be thinking, I already have diabetes so what is the relevance of telling me the effect of sugars and starches in increasing the risk of diabetes? It is a reasonable question. The point is, of course, that type 2 diabetes can be reversed, and in order to reverse the process it is important to understand what might have contributed to it in the first place. We know that eating too many calories causes people to gain weight, and that this increases the risk of diabetes. So part of reversing the process is to lose weight. However, learning that a high consumption of both sugars and some starches increases the risk of diabetes tells us that in order to reverse this process it would be a good idea to limit consumption of these particular carbohydrates. Which brings us to what has become quite the contentious issue in recent years: whether people with diabetes should be following a low-carbohydrate diet.

To many of us, reducing carbohydrates seems like plain common sense, yet the medical profession operates on what is termed 'evidence-based practice'. That is, before changing an approach to a condition or treatment protocol, there needs to be evidence that the change is beneficial. This usually takes the form of clinical trials. The trouble with lifestyle changes is that, unlike drugs, their effects are both complex and variable and depend hugely on many other factors – not least the motivation of the person making the changes. So studies, which compare one diet with another, may not always show clear-cut results. However, in recent years, a number of studies have come up with some interesting findings that we will look at now.

First of all we will examine the evidence that restricting carbohydrates is a good idea in people without diabetes. In 2012 a meta-analysis (where the results of multiple studies are compared) was published that looked at the results of 17 different studies into the effects of a low-carbohydrate diet on 1,141 people with obesity. This analysis showed that a low-carbohydrate diet was associated with significant reductions in weight (on average 7kg), waist circumference, blood pressure, fasting glucose levels, insulin levels and a rise in HDL (good) cholesterol.[8] One study showed that a low-carbohydrate diet was associated with greater weight loss and better cholesterol levels than a low-fat diet. Although termed a low-carbohydrate diet, in this study it was in fact a moderately restricted diet with 40 per cent of all calories from carbohydrates. In the low-fat diet 50 per cent of calories came from carbohydrates. Interestingly this study also looked at a Mediterranean diet with around 50 per cent calories from carbohydrate, but which included poultry and fish instead of red meat, and with added olive oil and nuts. In the short term this led to only small weight loss, but after two years, the results were similar to the low-carbohydrate diet group.[9]

So it appears that a restricted carbohydrate diet can work for obese people without diabetes, but what about for people with diabetes? A study in Australia looked at 100 people with poorly controlled type 2 diabetes who were following a standard diabetic diet in which 60 per cent of calories came from carbohydrates and 20 per cent from fat. The subjects then switched to a diet with 42 per cent calories from carbohydrate and an extra 15 per cent from 'healthy' polyunsaturated fats (olive oil and nuts) in addition to their usual fat intake. After 10 weeks on this diet there were significant reductions in body weight, fasting blood glucose, glycosylated haemoglobin (HbA1c) and cholesterol levels.[10]

Another study looked at a high-carbohydrate diet and one with less carbohydrates and more monounsaturated fats to compare their effects on diabetic control and on liver fat content. In this study the lower carbohydrate diet (despite containing more fat) led to better diabetic control and a significant reduction in liver fat.[11] A study from Japan asked people with poorly controlled type 2 diabetes to avoid carbohydrates at dinner (if their HbA1c was less than 75mmol/mol or 9 per cent), or at breakfast and dinner (if their HbA1c was above 75mmol/mol or 9 per cent). They could otherwise eat whatever they liked. After six months on this carbohydrate-restricted diet, both body weight and HbA1c levels fell significantly as did LDL-cholesterol levels. There were also significant reductions in both subcutaneous fat (fat under the skin), and crucially visceral fat (fat around the organs in the abdomen).[12] And these results were obtained just by removing carbohydrates from one or two meals a day.

At the further end of the scale are studies that have looked at very low-carbohydrate diets. A recent study from Germany looked at obese people with poorly controlled type 2 diabetes who were asked to follow a very low-carbohydrate diet (20g per day) for two months, with no other restrictions on what they could eat. After two months they could increase their carbohydrate intake. In this study they also took liraglutide (Victoza) injections. After six months the average HbA1c of the group fell from 9.0 per cent to 6.7 per cent, their body weight fell from 116kg to 101kg, again with big falls in LDL-cholesterol levels.[13]

These recent studies confirm that:

1. Reducing carbohydrates in the diet helps improve diabetes control and body weight
2. Reducing carbohydrates in the diet is also associated with less fat in the liver and lower LDL-cholesterol levels
3. These changes even occur if more fat is taken in the diet instead of carbohydrate

I have witnessed the same outcome in many of my patients since I started recommending carbohydrate restriction a few years ago. The effect of changing the diet in this way is far more dramatic than any medication, including insulin. And some people, who had been on insulin for many years to treat their type 2 diabetes, have even been able to come off it altogether. Taken together, these studies suggest that a lowered carbohydrate diet may be more effective in reversing diabetes by reducing fat content in the liver. The conclusion here is that for people who are overweight and have type 2 diabetes, and are therefore insulin resistant, the main culprit in the diet is likely to be eating too many carbohydrates.

We discussed earlier how low-fat, high-carbohydrate diets became the norm for healthy eating recommendations, and the more I read into the science of it, the more I am convinced that this has been a terrible mistake. So many people, including relatives of mine, focus on eating low-fat foods: consuming yoghurt with next to no fat in it (which frankly tastes disgusting) or low-fat cheese (which tastes like soap). Of course the low-fat 'healthy option' message is supported by a whole industry designed to take natural foods and turn them into something unnatural – often adding sugar for taste (remember: low fat equals low taste). Yet we have all collectively missed the point. We have had 40 years of low-fat recommendations, and a plethora of marketed low-fat foods, but over the same period the obesity epidemic has considerably worsened. Maybe our language doesn't help since the noun for the nutrient 'fat' is the same as the adjective describing someone who is overweight; perhaps subconsciously we link the two.

Increasingly the evidence points to carbohydrate as being an important contributing factor in people becoming overweight and getting fatty liver, which leads to diabetes. You may have heard of the French pâté, foie gras that is made from the livers of geese that have been force-fed to increase the fat content of their liver. What do you think they are fed on to bring this about? Carbohydrates!

So why are carbohydrates so bad? There are two important reasons: first, as we have learnt, the body turns all carbohydrates into sugars that increase blood glucose levels, making diabetes harder to control; second, and perhaps more importantly in the longer term, carbohydrates stimulate the pancreas to secrete insulin, and insulin is the body's main hormone that promotes the storage of fat – under the skin, in the abdomen, in the liver and just about everywhere else. The more insulin produced, the more fat is stored. The more fat stored in the liver, the more the body becomes resistant to insulin (as we learnt in chapter 2); the more insulin resistance, the more glucose levels rise, and the more insulin has to be produced – on and on in a vicious circle. Insulin also drives hunger, so when you eat carbohydrates you will produce insulin, which may well make you feel hungry again after a couple of hours. Fat and protein, on the other hand, are much better at satisfying hunger, meaning you can go for longer without eating – so you eat fewer calories and lose weight.

I recently had a very vivid personal experience of this when my wife and I were staying in a hotel before a 300-mile drive. I got a good deal at the hotel but it was room-only and rather than pay a huge amount for breakfast, we ate some cereal in the room before an early start. By mid-morning I was really quite hungry and had a couple of biscuits. At lunchtime we thought we would stop for a proper meal but were in a small town where we could only park for 30 minutes, and the only 'fast food' available at the place we chose was a panini and very nice it was too. However, three hours later I was very hungry again, but with still little time available, the best I could find in the service area was a slice of pizza. We popped in to see some relatives on the way home (and for a bite to eat) and they gave me bread and cheese. When we got home two hours later I was still hungry, despite seeming to have been eating all day. The reason? Every single meal was predominantly carbohydrate, leading to release of insulin, triggering more hunger. With my normal breakfast (based on Greek yoghurt) and lunch (soup or salad) I don't begin to feel peckish until late afternoon. Not only did my day of carbohydrate snacking prove to me the problem with eating carbs, it also highlighted how difficult it is to eat more healthily and with less carbs when you are on the move.

So, eating more carbs tends to increase appetite, calorie intake and hence weight. Is it any wonder therefore that through following the standard advice of a high-carbohydrate diet, type 2 diabetes was seen to be an inexorably progressive disease, characterised by increasing weight, worse glucose control, eventually leading to the need for insulin?

Yet with a simple change to the diet, whether it is my first-aid kit described earlier, or missing out carbs for one meal a day as in the Japanese study, you can begin to turn round this once-thought 'irreversible' condition, and set yourself on course to reverse your diabetes.

So cutting out some carbohydrates is a good first start to reversing your diabetes. As this will reduce calorie intake, it will in itself lead to some weight loss, as long as the carbohydrates are not replaced with extra fat or protein. Eating less carbohydrate-containing food will also help stabilise blood glucose levels. As discussed before, any change to your diet has to be permanent, so it has to be something that is not so drastic you start craving for foods you really like.

HOW MANY CARBS SHOULD I EAT?

If you search for low-carbohydrate diets online you will find all manner of diets on offer. My one piece of advice at this stage is not to go for any of them, and to generally steer clear of very low-carbohydrate diets, such as the Atkins diet, for three main reasons:

1. By reducing carbohydrate intake to less than 20g per day you will necessarily exclude all sorts of healthy nutrients; this could lead to nutritional deficiencies
2. These diets often suggest eating a high amount of fat, which may not in itself be very healthy
3. Such a very low-carbohydrate diet is rarely sustainable in the long term

Mostly, I favour a low-carbohydrate approach, which for most people would mean an intake of around 100g of carbohydrate per day. However, rather than trying to calculate your daily intake, I would start by experimenting with the choice of lower carbohydrate alternatives for your current meals. As we have seen from the studies I have quoted, in many cases reducing carbs also reduces calories and should help you lose weight as well as achieve better diabetes control.

Practical steps to reduce carbohydrate in your diet

In the next chapters I will look at different types of food in detail, but my 10-minute consultation on reducing carbohydrates goes something like this:

◆ What do you generally eat for breakfast?
◆ For lunch?
◆ For your evening meal?
◆ For snacks?

Typical answers will include cereal and toast for breakfast, perhaps with orange juice, a sandwich or baguette for lunch, maybe with a packet of crisps and an apple or banana for a snack, or maybe digestive biscuits. Followed by a variety of meals in the evening that usually includes potatoes, rice or pasta, which are all carbohydrates of course.

My first suggestion is to avoid cereals at breakfast and to try a breakfast based on eggs (boiled, poached or scrambled, with or without one slice of toast), or natural yoghurt. I find Greek yoghurt nicer (it is up to 10 per cent fat!) mixed with a handful of nuts or seeds and perhaps some oats. And, please, no fruit juice.

Lunch could be a home-made soup (avoiding starchy vegetables like potatoes and parsnips) or a salad, and while the evening meals can include carbohydrate, the carbs (bread, rice, potato or pasta) should occupy just a small corner of the plate, while filling up most of the plate with green vegetables or salad. Or try a meal with just meat and vegetables. So, as a rule, it is best to avoid meals based on carbohydrates such as potato or pasta bake, macaroni cheese, pizza or rice dishes. But enjoy them now and again, and accept your glucose will rise quite high afterwards.

For snacks, an apple, tangerine, peach, plum or pear are fine (i.e. any small 'round' fruit you can fit in the palm of your hand). Berries are also low in sugar. It is best to avoid eating bananas (unless a small one), pineapple or melon on a regular basis. Try to make up your five-a-day from vegetables rather than fruit. But you could also try a handful of nuts, which contain hardly any carbohydrates, but contain plenty of healthy fats.

With only this modest information to hand, many of my patients have achieved weight loss and much better control of their diabetes – without additional medication and without more detailed dietary advice. What is interesting is that by following this advice, people often find they are eating more fresh and natural foods, and less processed foods. Which will also mean eating less sugar and salt as they are to be found in worrying quantities in just about every type of processed foods.

PORTION SIZE

It is well established that over the years, portion sizes have increased. This not only applies to pre-prepared food but also, as food has become more available and affordable, to home-served foods. The old 'regular' serving of French fries in fast-food restaurants is now deemed to be a 'small' serving (if it exists at all); confectionery bars have grown larger (although in recent years there has been some reversal of this trend) and muffins and cookies are now often big enough to share. By now, it will be obvious that we don't actually need all this extra food. Whereas in previous generations the challenge was to get enough to eat, now the challenge is to limit what we eat. There are certain foods, such as green vegetables, that do not need to be limited (this will be explained in more detail in chapter 10), but in the context of controlling blood glucose levels, limiting carbohydrates is essential. As a general rule, I would suggest aiming for no more than about 30g of carbohydrate with each meal. It may be that certain individuals can manage more than this without adversely affecting their blood glucose level – and in chapter 13, we will learn how you can check how much your body can manage by measuring blood glucose levels before and after meals. Now this doesn't mean that you have to eat carbohydrates with every meal, and, as we saw earlier in this chapter, it is possible to survive very well (and improve blood glucose control) by having a very low-, or no, carbohydrate meal for one or two meals a day. On the other hand, you may occasionally have a larger portion of carbohydrates, as a special treat for example. However, this will likely cause a rise in blood glucose levels over the next few hours.

If you take insulin or a sulfonylurea tablet to control your diabetes, it is important that you eat and drink roughly the same amount of carbohydrate each day (unless you inject insulin with each meal), as otherwise there is a risk of hypoglycaemia, and learning how to assess and control your carbohydrate intake will help achieve more stable control. The table overleaf gives examples of different portion sizes of carbohydrates for different meals. This is not an exhaustive list, but is aimed at giving you an idea of how much a certain amount of carbohydrate looks like. I am very grateful to Chris Cheyette for providing this information, and would recommend his *Carbs & Cals* book (or its smartphone app)[14] as a very useful resource to help you learn more detail about carbohydrate portion size.

You'll find three examples of meals for each type and carbohydrate content. The carbohydrate-containing part of the meal is shown in **bold**. Note how some snacks (e.g. a flapjack) can contain 50g of carbohydrate, whereas some main meals (such as shepherd's pie) might only contain 20g.

GLYCAEMIC INDEX AND GLYCAEMIC LOAD

We have established that avoiding high-carbohydrate meals will help. This does not mean you should avoid carbohydrate altogether, however, as that can make your diet rather boring and increase the likelihood of missing out on some essential vitamins and minerals. What is important though is that wherever possible the

EXAMPLES OF MEALS OF DIFFERENT CARBOHYDRATE CONTENT

Grams Carbohydrate	Breakfast	Lunch
10 or less	1. 1 whole grapefruit with or without sweetener 2. Natural yoghurt (60g) with strawberries (80g) 3. 2 egg omelette with mushrooms, peppers	1. Mackerel salad with beetroot and horseradish 2. Vegetable soup (no potatoes) 3. Chicken salad
20	1. 4 small breakfast **pancakes** with bacon and cherry tomatoes 2. Scrambled egg on 1 slice thick **toast** 3. **Branflakes** (20g) with **milk**	1. Small slice **quiche** (100g) with salad 2. Smoked salmon on ½ **bagel** 3. 3 **Ryvita** with low-fat cream cheese
30	1. **All Bran** (40g) with **milk** 2. 2 slices medium **toast** with peanut butter 3. **Eggs benedict**	1. **Tomato soup** (1 tin) 2. Medium **wholegrain roll** with sliced turkey and salad 3. 3 bean **wrap**
40	1. Breakfast **pancakes** 2. 2 **Oatibix** with **milk** 3. No added sugar **muesli** (50g) with **milk**	1. Ham salad **sandwich** 2. **Cous cous** salad 3. 1 tin of **mushroom soup** with 2 medium slices wholegrain **bread**
50	1. 2 slices thick **toast** with **jam** 2. Large bowl **porridge** made with **milk** (350g) 3. **Croissant** with **marmalade** and glass **orange juice**	1. **Baked beans** on **toast** 2. 6 pieces of **sushi** 3. **Pasta** salad

Dinner	Snack
1. Tuna steak with steamed vegetables 2. Vegetable and bean stew. 3. Prawn stir fry with pineapple pieces	1. Apple 2. Plain popcorn (20g) 3. Almonds (30g)
1. **Shepherd's pie** (200g) with vegetables 2. Chilli con carne with **nachos** (20g) 3. Steak with grilled field mushroom and **new potatoes** (100g)	1. Medium **banana** 2. **Houmous** and vegetable sticks 3. Cereal bar
1. **Lasagne** (225g) with salad 2. Chicken stir fry with **egg noodles** (80g) 3. Baked salmon with small **jacket potato** and vegetables	1. **Coffee & walnut cake** (50g) 2. **Hot cross bun** 3. 2 scoops **vanilla ice cream**
1. Mushroom **risotto** (240g) 2. Chicken & broccoli **pasta** (340g) 3. Beef stew with 2 small **dumplings**	1. Malt loaf (60g) 2. Mince pie (60g) 3. Dates (60g)
1. 2 slices deep-pan **pizza** 2. **Lentil curry** with **brown rice** (95g) 3. Tuna **pasta** bake (350g)	1. **Flapjack** (80g) 2. Large hot-**chocolate drink** 3. Medium-sized **Easter egg** (100g)

carbohydrate eaten should have as little effect on blood glucose levels as possible.

This is where the concept of glycaemic index (GI) comes in. Some foods are absorbed very quickly which, in turn, causes the glucose level in the blood to rise sharply – these food types are termed high GI foods; other types of food that are absorbed more slowly are termed low GI foods. The glycaemic index of glucose itself is 100. The GI of orange juice is 50, which means that its effect on the blood glucose level is equivalent to half the effect of eating glucose. The table on pages 123–124 shows the GI for a number of common foods. It can be seen, for example, that a baguette has a very high GI of 95, whereas rye bread has a GI of just 58. Similarly, boiled potatoes have a GI of 50, whereas a baked potato has a GI of 85. Using this information will help you learn how to still enjoy eating bread or potatoes – by choosing types that have a low GI.

The overall effect of a food type on your blood glucose level will not depend merely on its glycaemic index, but also on how much of it you eat. For example, a very small piece of baguette (high GI) will have a much smaller effect on blood glucose and insulin levels than a whole plateful of boiled potatoes (lower GI notwithstanding).

The concept of glycaemic load (GL) has been introduced to take into account the actual amount of each type of food that is typically eaten. The equation is:

▶ GL = GI/100 x weight of net carbohydrate in a standard portion.

However, if you eat more or less than a standard portion then the GL will obviously be quite different for you.

Rather than getting too bogged down in the calculations, the GL can be useful in helping to identify those foods you can eat without restriction. Here's an example: you could eat a whole punnet of strawberries with very little effect on your glucose level (although they have a GI of 40). Because strawberries have such a low-carbohydrate content, the overall GL is only 1. White (durum wheat) pasta, on the other hand, which has a similar GI of 44, has a much higher carbohydrate content and is eaten in larger quantity, so has a GL of 21. The table that follows (adapted from John Briffa's book *Escape the Diet Trap*) provides further examples of the GI and GL of common carbohydrate foods.

At the end of the day it is the total amount of carbohydrate that will affect your blood glucose levels. Therefore, the key message is to stick to small portions of low GI foods wherever possible and to avoid high GI foods as much as you can.

NAUGHTY BUT NICE

This section covers sweet foods such as cakes, biscuits, pastries, sweets, chocolate, ice cream and desserts. They all contain sugar and will have an effect on your glucose and insulin levels. Apart from sugar, they also contain fat and anything other than a small portion will have a high-calorie content.

These foods do not serve any nutritional purpose and, simply put, we do not need to eat them. In an ideal world they are best avoided completely, and if you do not have a sweet tooth this may well be the best and easiest option. However, they are often very tasty, and regularly feature as part of many social events, such as birthday celebrations, a meal out or an ice cream on a hot sunny day. So if you do have a sweet tooth and can't resist the Siren call of the ice-cream van, make the effort to learn the carbohydrate content of your favourite sweet foods and find out how much you can get away with without it having a big effect on your glucose levels. The *Carbs & Cals* book is again very useful for this purpose. This will tell you, for example, that you can enjoy a small ice cream or portion of banoffee pie and only consume around 20g of carbohydrates. However, if you are anything like me, restricting yourself to a small portion will require a huge amount of willpower. It is best not to have these foods in your house, but enjoy them now and again as a treat when you are eating out.

One tip I learned recently for chocolate lovers: have some really good-quality dark chocolate in the house, break it up into squares and keep it in a container. Not only does dark chocolate contain all sorts of chemicals that are good for you, but, unless you are a complete chocoholic, it is very difficult to eat a large quantity of it. It also has a much lower sugar content than milk chocolate and is consequently a lot less moreish.

GI AND GL OF COMMON CARBOHYDRATE FOODS

Food type	Glycaemic Index (GI)	Glycaemic Load (GL)
BREAD		
Baguette	95	15
White bread – wheat	70	10
Rye bread – wholemeal	58	8
PASTA/RICE		
Brown rice	55	18
Basmati rice	58	22
White rice	64	23
Pasta – durum wheat	44	21
Pasta – wholewheat	37	16
SWEET FOODS		
Digestive biscuit	59	10
Doughnut	76	17
Scone	92	7
Ice cream	61	8
Mars bar	65	26
BEVERAGES		
Orange juice	50	13
Coca cola	53	14
Tomato juice	38	4
BREAKFAST CEREALS		
All Bran	42	8
Cornflakes	81	21
Muesli	40-66	12

Food type	Glycaemic Index (GI)	Glycaemic Load (GL)
FRUIT		
Apple	38	6
Banana	52	12
Grapes	46	8
Peach	42	5
Pear	38	4
Figs (dried)	61	16
Sultanas	60	25
Strawberries	40	1
LEGUMES		
Baked beans	48	7
Butter beans	31	6
Chick peas	28	8
Kidney beans	28	7
Green lentils	30	5
VEGETABLES		
Peas	48	3
Parsnips	97	12
Baked potato	85	26
Boiled potato	50	12
Mashed potato	74	15
Chips	75	17
Carrots – raw	16	1
Carrots – cooked	58	3
Beetroot	64	5

CHAPTER 10

OTHER FOOD TYPES
AND DRINK

FAT

Fat has a bad name – literally. As a noun it describes a type of food, but the same word, as an adjective, describes someone who is overweight. And so it is easy to link the two and think that fat in food causes fat people.

The body uses fat for energy stores and to protect most of our internal organs; it is also used to store vitamins such as vitamin D. It is therefore necessary to have some fat in our diet. It is true that fat has more calories per gram than either carbohydrate or protein. One gram of fat has about eight calories, whereas one gram of carbohydrate has only four calories. However, this does not necessarily mean eating fat means eating more calories. It does, of course, depend on how much fat-containing food you eat. Most high-fat foods (such as butter, cheese or cream) are eaten in quite small portions and consequently will mean less calories on the plate or in a serving than a standard portion of carbohydrates. Even meat that we tend to think of as fatty, such as pork, also has a lot of protein and its total calorie content may be quite modest. For example, an average portion of rice or pasta may contain 50g carbohydrates and around 250 calories in total. That is more than six rashers of grilled bacon (240 calories) and not much less than a generous 125g serving of roast pork (269 calories).

Fat in itself is, therefore, not fattening just because it is fat. It is only fattening if it is the reason why you are eating too many calories. Fat slows down the movement of food through the gut, so that you feel fuller for longer. Hence it tends to satisfy the hunger, which can mean you can actually end up eating less overall. Fat also has the advantage that it does not stimulate the production of insulin, which is, as you know by now, the main 'fat-storage' hormone.

Of course it makes sense not to overindulge in fat, or any other type of food for that matter. However, be careful when buying food that is labelled as 'low fat'. Often it is quite high in sugar. Let us take the example of yoghurt:

Grams (per 100g)	Natural Greek yoghurt	Low-fat flavoured yoghurt	0 per cent fat flavoured yoghurt
Carbs (sugar)	6	13.5	9.3
Fat	9.2	3.2	0.1
Calories	120	98	59

Now although the 0 per cent fat yoghurt has fewest calories, it still has the equivalent of nearly two teaspoons of sugar in it – but not much else. It is therefore not much more than a thickened sweet drink. It is therefore unlikely to satisfy hunger and you may end up eating something else a short time later, cancelling out the benefit of the low calories in the yoghurt.

However, if we compare the natural Greek yoghurt with the standard low-fat fruit yoghurt, you will see that the calorie content is quite similar. Although the low-fat yoghurt has less fat, there is over twice as much sugar (nearly three teaspoonfuls). This will increase the blood glucose level more than the Greek yoghurt and will stimulate the pancreas to produce more insulin to bring it down again. The increased insulin will have two effects: it will stimulate the production of fat, and increase the appetite, again increasing the chance that you will get hungry a short while later.

Although the Greek yoghurt has the highest fat content, this fat is very useful in slowing the absorption of the glucose from the gut, meaning the blood glucose level will rise much more slowly. It also means you are likely to feel satisfied after a smaller portion, and so the total amount of calories you eat may be less than if you ate one of the other types. As it has the lowest sugar content, the pancreas will release less insulin leading to less fat being stored in the liver and less hunger afterwards.

You could try for yourself eating a portion of each of these three types of yoghurt and checking your blood glucose beforehand and two hours afterwards, and determining how hungry you feel after two hours. This experiment may help you decide that low fat is not necessarily the best option for someone with diabetes!

Some types of fat are positively good for you. Monounsaturated fat is found in olive oil, sunflower oil (and seeds) and various types of nuts. Nuts have a low-carbohydrate content and their fat content (comprising mainly healthy fats) satisfies the appetite – a handful of nuts is therefore a good snack food. The Mediterranean diet (see chapter 9) is rich in monounsaturated fats and has several health benefits. A major study, published in 2013, demonstrated that taking a Mediterranean diet was associated with a 30 per cent reduction in cardiovascular events (e.g. heart attacks or strokes) compared to a low-fat diet.[1] What is also overlooked or understated is that about half of the fat in meat is monounsaturated.

PROTEIN

Proteins are large biological molecules consisting of chains of amino acids, the main elements of which are carbon, hydrogen, oxygen, and nitrogen. They are vital biochemical components found in all animal life forms, having a role in almost every process in cells. Our metabolism relies on a variety of proteins in a group known as enzymes that catalyse biochemical reactions, such as the action of insulin. Proteins have a role in building and maintaining body structures such as cell shape (cytoskeleton) and muscles. Others are important in our immune responses and something called cell adhesions, which is the binding together of cells in a multi-cellular organism. But the human body itself cannot actually make (or more accurately synthesise) amino acids, so we must obtain them from our food. Protein is found in meat, fish, eggs and beans and when these foods are digested, just as starch is broken down into glucose, we break down the ingested protein into free amino acids which are then available to our metabolic pathways where they are used to make a wide variety of vital molecules.

Protein in a meal leads to a small increase in production of insulin and a hormone called glucagon. Glucagon, like insulin, is produced by the pancreas and has the opposite effect of insulin in that it that raises levels of glucose in the blood. The pancreas releases it when blood sugar levels fall too low by converting stores of glycogen in the liver to glucose, which is then released into the bloodstream. Insulin and glucagon act as a part of a feedback process keeping glucose levels stable. It can convert fat into glucose and this is good in terms of helping burn excess fat; the slight rise in blood glucose is not too much of a problem if your carbohydrate intake is reduced.

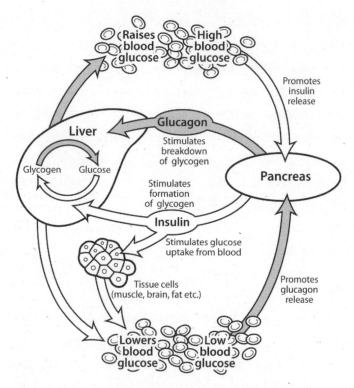

Illustration reproduced with the kind permission of the International Diabetes Federation, taken from The IDF Diabetes Atlas *(sixth edition)*

The body can also use amino acids to form glucose when glucose stores run out. This conversion requires energy, that is, it uses up calories, which in itself may help with weight loss.

Like fat, protein is very effective in satisfying the appetite and studies have shown that when people are asked to increase their protein intake they tend to eat fewer calories overall – again contributing to weight loss.

As protein is made of amino acids it makes the stomach more acidic. This has the effect of slowing the digestive process so that the stomach is fuller for longer – so you don't feel the need to eat so much. However, some authorities express concern that protein is harmful to the kidneys. While it is true that people with poor kidney function may need to restrict their protein intake, there is little evidence to suggest moderate protein intake is harmful to those with normal kidney function.

Meat and fish are good sources of protein, as are dairy products (milk, cheese and yoghurt) and eggs. In the good old days eggs were seen as a natural and healthy component of our diet, but the poor egg has had a very bad press over recent years. Because they are a natural source of cholesterol it was thought they were bad for our health; then there were various scares about eggs containing salmonella. We now recognise that high cholesterol levels result from obesity and insulin resistance more than anything else; in the UK salmonella has been eradicated as a result of vaccination of poultry. Eggs are now deemed to be safe and there are no restrictions on the amount of eggs we consume. Eggs are a low-calorie food (70–80 per egg when poached or boiled) and as they are high in protein tend to satisfy the appetite.

For vegetarians it is important to have an adequate intake of protein-rich pulses (such as kidney beans and lentils); nuts and seeds are also good sources of protein.

In summary, both protein and fat have their advantages, and if eaten in moderation are healthy alternatives to carbohydrates. As we read in chapter 8, man has evolved to live healthily on a variety of diets including those mainly based on fat and protein.

FRUIT, VEGETABLES, GRAINS AND NUTS

Fruit and vegetables are generally considered healthy and often lumped together in health messages. We are all aware of the recommendation to eat a minimum of five portions of fruit and vegetables every day, as explained in the following quote from the NHS UK Choices website:[2]

> *Eat lots of fruit and veg It's recommended that we eat at least five portions of different types of fruit and veg a day. It's easier than it sounds. A glass of 100 per cent unsweetened **fruit juice** can count as one portion, and vegetables cooked into dishes also count. Why not chop a **banana** over your breakfast cereal, or swap your usual mid-morning snack for some **dried fruit**?*
>
> *What counts towards 5 A Day?*
>
> *The following count towards your 5 A Day:*
> * *Fresh fruit and vegetables.*
> * *Frozen fruit and vegetables.*
> * *Tinned or canned fruit and vegetables. Buy the ones tinned in natural juice or water with no added sugar or salt.*

- *Dried fruit such as currants, dates, sultanas and figs.*
- *Fruit and vegetables cooked in dishes such as soups, stews or pasta dishes.*
- *A glass (150ml) of unsweetened 100 per cent fruit or vegetable juice. Juice counts as a maximum of one portion a day however much you drink. That is mainly because juice contains less fibre than whole fruits and vegetables.*
- *Smoothies. A smoothie containing all of the edible pulped fruit and/or vegetable may count as more than one portion, but this depends on how it is made. Smoothies count as up to a maximum of two portions per day.*
- *Beans and pulses. These only count as one portion a day no matter how many you eat. That is because they contain fewer nutrients than other fruits and vegetables.*
- *Fruit and vegetables in convenience foods such as ready meals and shop-bought pasta sauces, soups and puddings. Some ready-made foods are high in salt, sugar and fat so only have them occasionally or in small amounts. You can find the salt, sugar and fat content of ready-made foods on the label.*

The highlighted items are all high in sugar, yet are recommended as being a healthy option. A recent study conducted at University College of London resulted in newspaper headlines including this from the *Guardian* in April 2014: 'Fruit and vegetable intake: five a day may not be enough, scientists say. UCL study suggests increase in daily fruit and veg intake linked to lower chance of death from stroke and cancer.' It has been suggested that seven-a-day provides more benefit. However, the official recommendation for now remains at five-a-day. This is just as well, as I shudder to think of the consequences of people being encouraged to consume even more smoothies and fruit juice.

What becomes clear is that whatever criteria were used to determine what counts towards five-a-day, they certainly did not take into account the sugar content. And yet these high-sugar foods mean that many 'five-a-day' foods are really not ideal for a person with diabetes.

Now vegetables contain very little sugar and, in the case of leafy vegetables, very little starch, but they do contain plenty of vitamins and minerals and fibre – all good stuff. However, much of the above list relates to fruit in various forms. And what does fruit contain? Sugar. Now a lot of it is fructose, or fruit sugar, which by definition does not raise blood glucose levels. But it is still full of calories, and as we learned in chapter 9 causes its own problems. So, even no-added-sugar juice or tinned fruits are not a good idea. My own view is that fruit juice should not be included in the five-a-day list, unless taken in very small quantities, as most of the bits that make fruit healthy have been removed: a 200ml glass of orange juice contains 112 calories, 21g of sugar and only 0.1 g of fibre. A whole orange, on the other hand, only contains 45 calories and 9g of sugar while providing 2.3g of dietary fibre. Smoothies, also marketed as being full of goodness, are even worse. A review by the consumer organisation *Which?* found that they contain more calories per 100ml than Coca-Cola. Nearly half the smoothies contained 30g or more of sugar per 250ml, the equivalent of six teaspoons of sugar. They also found that nearly a third of consumers wrongly believe that the drinks contain two of the recommended five-a-day portions of fruit and vegetables, when they do not.[3]

For anyone wishing to reverse their diabetes, this message needs to be amended to steer people away from sugary foods. I would recommend avoiding fruit juices and smoothies completely and to never drink them to quench your thirst. I would also suggest avoiding dried fruit, except in very small quantities (e.g. a few raisins in some yoghurt) because when the water is removed to produce dried fruit, it leaves it with a very high sugar content. Tropical fruits such as bananas, pineapple and mangoes are also high in sugar and should not be eaten on a regular basis. Suitable fruits for someone with diabetes are berries (which have a very low sugar content) and apples, pears, peaches and small citrus fruits such as tangerines, i.e. whole fruit that you can hold in your hand.

Vegetables, on the other hand, contain much less sugar than fruit, but differ greatly in the amount of starch they contain, depending on the type. Starch is the carbohydrate used by plants to store energy and the most common form of carbohydrate in the human diet. It is therefore best to consider vegetables in four broad categories: 'fruit' vegetables; leafy vegetables; legumes (peas and beans); and root vegetables.

Salad vegetables, such as tomatoes, cucumber and red and green peppers, are in fact the fruits of the plant as they contain the seeds. However, they are generally eaten as vegetables. They all have quite low sugar content and can be eaten freely.

Leafy vegetables are generally from plants where we eat the green leaves that grow above ground. Examples include broccoli, cabbage, spinach, lettuce and cauliflower. These are all rich in fibre and vitamin C, with very low sugar or starch content, and can be eaten in unlimited quantities.

Root vegetables are those where we eat the roots such as all types of potatoes, carrots, turnips, parsnips and beetroots. These roots store energy for the plant that helps them to survive as they lie dormant over winter. Much of this energy is in the form of starchy carbohydrate and for this reason anyone with diabetes should eat root vegetables in moderation. Some, such as onions, carrots and swedes, are about 10 per cent carbohydrate, so a usual portion will contain very little carbohydrate. Potato and parsnips are nearer 20 per cent and should only be eaten in small quantities. Beetroot is 10 per cent carbohydrate, of which 7 per cent is sugar.

Legumes are a class of vegetable that produce beans that are either eaten alone (such as peas or broad beans) or together with their 'pods' such as French beans, runner beans or sugar snap peas. Their carbohydrate content varies considerably and so it is important to know which ones are high and which are low in carbohydrate.

Any that are eaten with their pods are low in carbohydrate and can be eaten freely. Split peas and chickpeas contain about 40 per cent and 50 per cent carbohydrate respectively, and are best avoided as they are often eaten in quite large quantities. Lentils and black-eye beans are better options, but still contain around 20 per cent carbohydrate; red kidney beans are only 7 per cent carbohydrate.

Garden peas are relatively low in carbohydrate; however, beware mushy peas that are very dense and can contain much more carbohydrate than you might think. Sweetcorn is strictly speaking a grain, but is often viewed as a vegetable similar to peas. However, it contains around 20 per cent carbohydrate and anything more than a small portion will increase your glucose level.

Grains are foods that come from wheat, rice, oats, barley or other cereal grains. They are rich in carbohydrates and all types of bread, pasta, rice and breakfast cereals fall into this category. Grains are classified either as wholegrains or refined grains. Wholegrains are recommended as they contain dietary fibre, iron and a number of B vitamins. Examples include wholemeal flour, brown rice or wholemeal pasta. Refined grains have been milled, a process that removes the fibre, iron and vitamins, to produce white flour, white rice or pasta. When the fibre is removed by way of the refining process, it increases the glycaemic index, meaning these products will have a greater effect on blood glucose levels. For people with diabetes, wholegrains are to be preferred. While many people enjoy wholemeal bread many find wholemeal pasta, for example, unappetising. Some people with irritable bowel syndrome may not be able to eat wholegrains that contain insoluble fibre. It is also important to remember that a large portion of rice or pasta will have a big effect on your glucose and insulin levels, regardless of the type. It is just that the wholemeal variety will lead to a more prolonged effect. The advice, therefore, is to eat and enjoy the types of bread, rice or pasta that you like, but to keep to small portions, especially if it is a refined type (e.g. white bread or rice).

NUTS AND SEEDS

We will consider nuts and seeds together, as their nutritional value is very similar. Nuts and seeds contain protein and healthy plant fat with relatively little carbohydrate. They are quite high in energy and so a small portion such as a handful of nuts is a good option for a snack and will satisfy hunger, but will have no significant effect on your blood glucose or insulin levels. Nuts or seeds can also be added to natural yoghurt to make a nutritious, unprocessed alternative to breakfast cereal. Beware, however, that even a moderate portion will contain many calories – a small 50g pack of peanuts, for example, contains nearly 300 calories.

To summarise: in order to help reverse your diabetes it is important not to lump all fruit and vegetables together, as current recommendations do. Focus on eating those that will have the least effect on your glucose or insulin levels, such as:

- Berries
- Leafy and salad vegetables
- Mange tout and French or runner beans

The following can be eaten in moderation:

- Apples, pears, citrus fruit, peaches
- Carrots and swedes
- Peas, lentils and kidney beans
- Seeds and nuts

And these should be eaten in small quantities only:

- Banana, pineapple, melon
- Potatoes, parsnips and chick peas
- Bread, rice, pasta and breakfast cereals

Fruit juice and smoothies should be avoided altogether. However, if you really enjoy these have a small glass and enjoy the texture and flavour. Don't drink them to quench your thirst or to satisfy hunger.

ANYONE FOR A DRINK?

Drinks are an important part of life and many are very enjoyable. However, strictly speaking, we only need one and that is water. Or perhaps two, if you include breast milk for babies.

Water is an essential part of our diet not least because our bodies consist of over 60 per cent water; we need to constantly replace the water used to drive chemical processes in our body, the water used in the production of sweat that helps keep us cool, and the water in our urine that removes waste. It is recommended that we drink at least 1.2 litres a day, which is six average-sized glasses or cups. It doesn't have to be plain water and can include other drinks such as tea and coffee, but it is important to ensure the drinks you choose will not make it more difficult to reverse your diabetes.

Water is undoubtedly the best drink for quenching thirst – it is cheap, natural and contains no calories. It is also good for you. In the UK we have no excuse for not drinking plenty of water – tap water is clean and safe. The situation is very different in many low-income countries, where tragically it is sometimes safer to drink bottled sugary drinks than water. It is a good idea to have a glass of water to hand at all times. Keeping well hydrated improves alertness and concentration and access to water in schools has been shown to improve cognitive function.[4] So many drinks contain sugar, that just by switching to drinking water, many people will reduce their calorie intake sufficiently to lose weight and significantly reduce their risk of developing diabetes. Indeed to encourage this, I coined the phrase 'Fight diabetes – drink water', which I think says it all.

Some people have told me they don't like drinking tap water and pay to buy bottled water or flavoured water. What a waste of money! Let me offer you a tip: buy some fresh lemons and limes, slice them neatly, lay the slices out on a plate and freeze them individually. They can then be stored in a container in your freezer and added to a glass of ordinary tap water – providing a natural flavouring as well as being an organic ice-cube! Drinking a glass of water before you eat is said by some to help you lose weight by making your stomach fuller so you feel you don't need to eat so much.

Tea and coffee are an important part of daily life. Green tea, especially, is said to have health benefits, but drinking too much caffeine (found in tea and coffee) is not a good idea as it can cause excessive stimulation of the heart. However, drinking a few cups of tea or coffee is unlikely to pose a problem. Unless you are partial to lattes made with full-fat milk (too many calories) or put heaped teaspoonfuls of sugar in every cup (too much sugar).

Caffeine itself has been shown to reduce the effect of insulin (i.e. increasing insulin resistance) by about 15 per cent.[5] Indeed, in the past, this property has led to caffeine being recommended for people taking insulin to help prevent their glucose level falling too low. I know of some patients who have stopped drinking coffee (or used decaffeinated coffee) and have found it led to a marked improvement in their blood glucose levels. Other studies have suggested that a moderate caffeine intake protects against type 2 diabetes. If you are trying to reverse your diabetes it is important to try and improve your insulin sensitivity, and if you habitually drink a lot of coffee, reducing it may help make a difference – it is certainly worth a try.

Other hot drinks, such as drinking chocolate or malted drinks, contain a significant amount of sugar. In their powdered form they contain around 80 per cent sugar. A standard serving of drinking chocolate may contain 12g sugar (equivalent to three teaspoons) and the milk contains another 12g. Powdered milkshake drinks, to be mixed with cold milk and generally marketed for children, contain about 18g of sugar per serving (plus the 12g in the milk). These will all raise blood glucose levels significantly in a person with diabetes.

I have covered fruit juices and smoothies earlier in this chapter, but in case you missed it, I really want to recommend that you avoid them, other than in very small quantities. For the same reason, all sugar-sweetened drinks, such as orange squash and fizzy (carbonated) drinks, should be avoided. If you must drink carbonated drinks then I would recommend consuming diet or no-added sugar varieties. Some people are anxious about the effects of artificial sweeteners – but when it comes to diabetes, I think the artificially sweetened varieties are far preferable to the sugar-sweetened ones.

We all know that too much alcohol is bad for our health and the guidelines on the amounts of alcohol consumption are the same for people with diabetes as those without it (up to 14 units for women and 21 for men each week). Many of us underestimate our alcohol consumption and over the years many drinks have become stronger than they used to be. For example, many wines are now 12–13 per cent alcohol compared to 10 per cent a few years ago, and the beers drunk today, such as continental lagers, are typically 5 per cent compared to 3 per cent in a traditional British bitter. Not only is excess alcohol bad for the liver, the heart and in fact just about every other part of the body, alcohol itself contains calories which can cause weight gain and all the problems that ensue from it.

For people with diabetes we also have to consider the effect of alcoholic drinks on blood glucose levels. Alcohol itself can have an effect of lowering blood glucose and for people treated with insulin in particular consumption of a large amount of alcohol can lead to glucose levels falling too low. For people with type 2 diabetes, the main concern is the effect of specific drinks in increasing glucose levels, and the calories (from both sugar and alcohol) in causing weight gain and fat accumulation.

Beer contains carbohydrate in the form of starch and a very small amount of sugar (in the form of maltose). The amount varies according to the type, but on average a pint of beer may contain about 10g of carbohydrate. Anything more than one pint will therefore have a definite effect in raising blood glucose levels. Cider is generally sweeter, up to 20g of sugar per pint, and is best avoided altogether. Most wine is generally low in carbohydrate with the exception of sweet white wine. Some liqueurs are very sweet: Baileys is about 20 per cent sugar and Amaretto 60 per cent! Anything other than a very small shot will definitely increase your glucose level. Spirits, on the other hand, are generally free from carbohydrate and will have no effect on raising your glucose level. However, they are often drunk with a sugar-containing mixer. Also beware that low-alcohol beers and wines generally have high-carbohydrate content.

In summary, I would recommend low-carb drinks such as dry white wine, red wine or spirits (without sweet mixers) in order to minimise the effect on blood glucose levels.

Type of drink with standard serving size (% alcohol by volume)	Grams of carbohydrate	Units of alcohol
Vodka: 25ml single measure (40%)	0	1
Gin, rum: 50ml double (40%) with slimline mixer	0	2
Cognac: 50ml double measure (40%)	0	2
Pilsner beer: 330ml bottle (5%)	0	2
White wine: 175ml regular glass (12.5%)	5	2
Red wine: 250ml large glass (15%)	5	4
Port, sherry, vermouth: 50ml glass (15–20%)	5	1
Beer: 1 pint (3–4%)	10	2

Other Food Types and Drink

Type of drink with standard serving size (% alcohol by volume)	Grams of carbohydrate	Units of alcohol
Lager: 330ml bottle (5%)	10	2
Liqueur: (Baileys Irish Cream, Tia Maria) 50ml	15	1
Stout (Guinness): 1 pint (4%)	15	2
Cider: 1 pint (5%)	20	2½
Bacardi Breezer, Smirnoff Ice: 275ml bottle (5%)	25 – 30	1½
Double Vodka Red Bull	25	2
Vintage cider: 500ml bottle (8%)	40	4
Low-alcohol beer: 330ml bottle (less than 1%)	20	trace
Low-alcohol wine: 175ml glass (less than 1%)	20	trace
Cola, lemonade, fruit juice: 150ml as mixer	15	0
Red Bull: 200ml can	25	0
J20: 330ml bottle	35	0
Mineral water, soda water, slimline or diet drinks	0	0

CHAPTER 11

MINERALS, VITAMINS AND SUPPLEMENTS

You won't be surprised to learn that I have read many books that offer diet plans for people with type 2 diabetes. Increasingly, they also offer the prospect of reversing diabetes. While they share the common goal of achieving control (or reversal) of diabetes by changing the diet, their recommendations vary massively. What matters most is that the diet leads to weight loss, that it stabilises blood glucose levels, and it is sustainable in the long term. To be sustainable you need to be able to eat a variety of foods that you enjoy, and to my mind, that means that there shouldn't be too many restrictions. The diet should also provide all the nutrients you need, including vitamins and minerals. I have seen one plan, for example, that advocates a high-carbohydrate vegan diet, together with a whole host of vitamins or supplements to replace those lost by excluding so many natural foods. Very low-carbohydrate diets also risk leading to mineral deficiencies.

The generally accepted advice on supplements is that if you eat a healthy, balanced diet then you should not need to take additional vitamins or minerals. A diet based on fresh meat and fish, fruit and vegetables, nuts or seeds and appropriate portions of grains will provide most of the vitamins and minerals that you need. I am not a nutritionist, nor do I have much experience of the use of supplements for the treatment of diabetes (and cannot comment on the claims made for many supplements); however, I am aware of scientific research that suggests some supplements may help reduce glucose levels, and therefore could be directly relevant to the goal of reversing your diabetes. These are chromium, cinnamon and vitamin D.

CHROMIUM

The chemical element chromium, which is a steel-grey metal and a trace element in human bodies, has been shown in several scientific studies to have an effect on reducing insulin resistance – a key goal in reversing diabetes. It is thought to have a role in helping insulin bind to its receptor on cell walls, which is the key (literally) to allowing glucose to enter cells. Chromium is found in foods such as meat, liver and wholegrains; however, most of the chromium is removed during refining processes, especially in the production of white flour. A review of over 40 studies showed that supplements of chromium improved diabetes control and that the best effects were seen with chromium picolinate at doses of 400 to 1000mcg a day.[1, 2] There is no evidence that chromium supplementation is harmful.

CINNAMON

Cinnamon is obtained from the bark of trees from the *Cinnamomum* family, and has been used as a spice since biblical times. One study of people with type 2 diabetes, treated with sulfonylurea tablets, showed that taking a small dose (as little as 1g per day) of cinnamon cassia led to a significant reduction in fasting levels of both blood glucose and cholesterol.[3] A recent review of several laboratory studies found that another variety (*Cinnamon zeylanicum*) was associated with a number of beneficial changes.[4] Some nutritionists recommend taking 3g (a teaspoonful) of cinnamon a day to help people with diabetes reduce their glucose levels.

VITAMIN D

Vitamin D is more accurately described as a hormone; it helps the body maintain the correct level of calcium in the blood. For vitamin D to be effective it needs to undergo a chemical change in the skin and the catalyst for the change is sunlight. Adequate exposure to the sun is important to maintain vitamin D levels. Modern man (and woman) spends most of the time indoors or in the car. When outside in the UK, the chances of being able to expose our skin to the sunlight (a warm, sunny day) are few and far between. It is hardly surprising, therefore, that vitamin D deficiency is quite a common problem and can be especially problematic in people with darker skin.

A number of studies have suggested that a lack of vitamin D is associated with the increased risk of insulin resistance and type 2 diabetes. Some studies[5] have shown that taking vitamin D can help reduce insulin resistance, whereas others have failed to show any benefit. There is certainly no harm in taking a small supplement of vitamin D (e.g. 25mcg a day).

In summary, if you are interested in taking nutritional supplements you may wish to consider taking one of the above. I would not recommend any others as long as you have a good balanced diet. It is very important that your doctor is aware of any supplements you are taking.

CHAPTER 12

IT'S TIME TO GET MORE ACTIVE

In chapter 4 we discussed how type 2 diabetes is initially managed by 'diet and exercise'. So far we have concentrated on the diet part of this duo: in this chapter we will look at the exercise part.

Exercise is recommended for people with diabetes because it has been shown that it helps reduce blood glucose levels. Regular aerobic exercise, such as running or 'cardiovascular' workouts, has been shown to reduce HbA1c by around 7mmol/mol (0.7 per cent), whereas anaerobic or resistance exercise (such as weight training) by around 5mmol/mol (0.5 per cent). Combining the two does slightly better, resulting in a 8mmol/mol (0.8 per cent) improvement. However, when one looks at the duration of exercise per week, it has been shown that at least 150 minutes (per week) is required to achieve meaningful improvements in HbA1c. Anything less than this will make little difference.[1, 2]

Since the diabetes prevention studies of the early 2000s, the standard advice has been that you should aim to take a 30-minute brisk walk at least five times a week, in order to achieve the 150-minute goal. The emphasis is on the 'brisk', meaning the exercise has to raise your heart rate and bring you out in a bit of a sweat. For many people, especially those of us who might be described as overweight and essentially unfit, the idea of exercise can seem quite challenging, possibly frightening. Although a brisk walk may be seen as a less challenging task than a vigorous workout at the gym, attempting a cross-country run, or swimming 20 lengths of the local pool, a weekly routine of five brisk walks a week is probably unrealistic for someone who is not used to any form of exercise. This may well explain why, even in the large trials, the target of 150 minutes of exercise a week was never met; the actual amount achieved averaged nearer to 60 minutes.

A more recent study has looked at the effect of exercise in conjunction with diet advice in people recently diagnosed with type 2 diabetes. Encouraging people to undertake 150 minutes of exercise each week did not, in fact, lead to any significant benefits above the effect of dietary advice alone, suggesting that, at least in the early stages of diabetes, dietary changes are the most important.[3] It is known that exercise can increase hunger, and it is possible that eating afterwards could have reversed the benefits of this type of exercise. However, there is increasing evidence that there are two other factors to be taken into account, rather than just the process of exercise alone. These are activity levels and sedentary time.

One of the earliest studies that showed the beneficial effect of exercise did not look at encouraging moderate or vigorous exercise; rather it examined the activity levels associated with the participants' employment. In the 1950s a research team looked at the health of two groups of workers in London: bus drivers (who spent several hours sat behind the steering wheel) and bus conductors, who in London in those days would run up and down the stairs found at the back of double-decker buses all day long. The study also looked at postmen, who spent much of their day walking, and telephone switchboard operators who, like the bus drivers, were seated during their working hours. They found that the more active workers (postmen and bus conductors) had lower death rates from heart disease than their less active colleagues.[4] And this leads us to conclude that walking, as part of your job, is healthier than sitting down all day. The beneficial effects of this type of occupational activity were emphasised by a recent study from Denmark, in which active healthy volunteers were persuaded to reduce their activity from over 10,000 steps a day to less than 1,500. After just two weeks they had already demonstrated evidence of higher blood insulin levels and a significant increase in abdominal fat.[5]

More recent research has examined the impact of so-called sedentary time. In one study over 500 adults with newly diagnosed type 2 diabetes were asked to wear an accelerometer, a wearable device that measures activity levels. The subjects also had various other measurements performed to assess their overall metabolic health. The accelerometers were analysed to determine how long the subjects spent being inactive. The study concluded that the longer the time spent sitting each day, the greater the level of insulin in the blood and of insulin resistance. This inactive time was also associated with an increase in waist circumference of 1.9cm (about ¾ of an inch), and with a reduction in healthy HDL cholesterol – both known consequences of insulin resistance.[6] So it is possible that the more time we spend sitting down, the more likely we are to develop type 2 diabetes. Indeed, this was the conclusion of a meta-analysis of a number of studies that looked at the effect of time spent watching TV and health. This showed that, on average, for every two hours spent watching television each day, the risk of developing diabetes increased by 20 per cent, and the risk of death from all causes increased by 13 per cent. Incredibly, people who spent five hours a day watching television had a 50 per cent increased risk of developing diabetes.[7] Of course, it may not just be the sitting down that is bad for your health; unhealthy food eaten while watching television may also contribute. Another way of looking at it is to argue that in some cases people are watching too much television because they are overweight and less mobile in the first place. Nevertheless, even taking these factors into account, the research suggests that two hours a day watching television increases the risk of diabetes by 13 per cent.

If watching more television increases the risk of diabetes, then you would hope that reducing the amount of time spent watching television would have the opposite effect. Support for this comes from a small study from the United States in which a group of 36 overweight people (BMIs of between 25 and 50) who self-reported a three hours per day average television viewing habit were randomly split into a control group and an intervention group. The intervention group were asked to reduce their television viewing time by 50 per cent. After three weeks, the intervention group were found to have significantly increased their energy expenditure (measured using an accelerometer) and to have lost some weight.[8]

You may think that doing the recommended 150 minutes of exercise a week would mean spending less time in front of the television. Well, it isn't necessarily the case. A study in Australia looked at data from over 4,000 people who all did at least 150 minutes each week of moderate to vigorous exercise. They were asked how long they spent watching television, and it was found that even in this 'healthy' group, a longer time spent in front of the television was associated with a bigger waist circumference, higher blood pressure and higher blood glucose levels.[9] The authors of this study described such people as 'active couch potatoes'! This type of study is very important as it emphasises that the good that comes from exercise can be undone by too much sitting down.

Even if one doesn't watch television, modern life means that long periods of sedentary time are inevitable for many people, for example those whose job involves driving or sitting at a desk. What can these people do to try and preserve their health? Studies have looked at the effect of 'breaks' in sedentary time. The study in the 500 people who wore accelerometers showed that those who interrupted their sedentary time, even for as short a time as one minute, had a smaller waist circumference. This was confirmed in another study that showed that having more breaks during sedentary time was associated with a reduction in waist circumference, body weight and blood glucose levels, compared to subjects who did not interrupt their time sitting down.[10] There are a number of possible reasons for this, including the fact that the act of standing, even for a short time, uses significantly more energy than sitting down.

How we get to work also has an effect on our health. A recent study from London looked at the health of over 20,000 people from the UK who took part in a national survey, and described how they got to work. Any type of 'active travel' to work (walking, cycling or using public transport) was associated with a lower likelihood of being overweight. Walking and cycling were both associated with a lower likelihood of having diabetes.[11] However, the message is that you don't have to walk or cycle all the way to work to benefit. As most people using public transport have to walk to and from the bus stop or train station each day, using a bus or train is actually better for you than driving.

I had my own experience of this when, many years ago, I worked at a hospital in London. I had to walk to my local station to catch the train, and, after a 30-minute train journey, walk from London's Waterloo Station to the hospital. In total I was walking nearly two miles every day. I then moved jobs to a hospital where I had to drive for 90 minutes each day to get to work. This increased my sedentary time by an hour and reduced my exercise time by 40 minutes every working day. Guess what happened – my weight began to increase.

So what does all this mean for someone wanting to reverse his or her diabetes? The evidence clearly shows that physical inactivity, and in particular long periods sitting down, increases the risk of gaining weight and of developing diabetes. The studies also demonstrate that regular physical activity such as walking or cycling to work helps prevent diabetes. More strenuous exercise can improve diabetes control if it is undertaken for at least 150 minutes each week, as long as one is careful not to undo its effect by eating afterwards. Reducing sedentary time (by spending less time watching television or working at a computer, for example) can help with weight loss, and possibly help reverse diabetes, and breaking up long periods of sedentary time by simply getting up for a stretch actually helps reduce the harmful effects of sedentary periods.

Many studies of people with diabetes show that the most important factor in controlling (or reversing) diabetes is dietary change, and that the effects of exercise really benefit those who have a healthy diet in place. So the priority must be to adopt some of the dietary changes outlined in this book, rather than simply signing up for a gym membership. However, the evidence is that the changes to your lifestyle that increase your activity levels will certainly be beneficial. Not only will being more active help reverse the diabetes disease process by reducing insulin and glucose levels in the blood, and help reduce your weight and waist size, it will also protect against high blood pressure and heart disease. It will also make you feel better and more energetic and possibly more in control of your diabetes. Remember that any changes have to be sustainable, and that means they and you have to be realistic. The most effective changes are ones that will cause you to increase your activity as part of routines and behaviours (like using public transport) in your daily life, rather than trying to stick to an exercise regime just for the sake of exercising.

As far as we know our ancient ancestors didn't go to the gym or go jogging! They kept healthy by using their bodies for the purpose for which they were designed (or evolved). Humans are designed to walk, and walking forms the most accessible form of exercise for everyone (with the exception, of course, of those with a physical disability that makes walking difficult). An obvious target for increased activity is simply to walk more; and use the car less. The UK Department for Transport estimates that one car journey in five is for a distance of less than one mile! Consider setting yourself this simple target: only use the car for journeys greater than one mile. That would mean walking to the shop round the corner for the extra pint of milk. If you work within two miles of your home think about walking to work. It might be a struggle at first, but as your fitness increases you will find it gets easier (even pleasurable); you will be accomplishing a significant amount of exercise and saving money as a bonus!

In the past if somebody had said to me that walking was an effective way to improve your fitness, I would have been sceptical. I had always understood that fitness and conditioning training involved a lot of hard yards and effort. Now I have come to realise that walking plays a fundamental role in what is called conditioning training. It's a great starting point to build up your confidence, especially if you have not been involved in any sort of training or fitness-related activities for a while – or if you have never been that keen on sport in the first place. Walking will allow you to start achieving small, short-term goals and aid in measurable weight loss.

Walking is a great stepping-stone towards future fitness; don't underestimate its value. If you can manage three or four brisk walks a week with a two-hour walk at the weekend, you will notice a major improvement in your fitness after six weeks.

To begin with, you can also take it at your own pace without the likelihood of seriously injuring yourself, and then start to increase the difficulty by either walking for longer, or faster, up steeper gradients or even carrying modest weights.

The benefits of walking include:

▶ improving your cardiovascular efficiency
▶ helping prevent osteoporosis
▶ improving your all-round mobility
▶ and it's perfect for those of more advanced years or for people returning to fitness after a period of inactivity

And of course walking provides an excuse to enjoy the great outdoors. During the first time you tackle a country ramble with heavy boots and a backpack, you may look forward to the end of the day so you can relax, soak your feet and have a hot bath; after a few walks, you will notice that the aches in your back, hips and neck have diminished, as the 'Longer, Lower, Regular' nature of country walking starts working on your body. 'Longer, Lower, Regular' is an uncomplicated and memorable way of understanding how to condition your body for better endurance (all-round fitness). Basically, you train for longer periods at low intensity and as regularly as you can while staying out of the red zone or high-intensity work.[12]

In the gym, the treadmill is a standard piece of equipment, but like so many bits of kit, most people have no idea how to use it; you will often see people pounding away at a rate of knots or looking like they're on the Great March and apparently close to exhaustion.

Always start at a sensible intensity – 5km an hour is good for most people – and then gradually build it up to a brisk walk, before increasing the gradient (again gradually) so that more muscle groups come into play, including your back and shoulders.

Cycling is another terrific alternative to driving and may be more suitable for people who are overweight as the bicycle helps support your body – especially the joints, which means you can comfortably exercise for longer. Cycling also enables you to travel faster and further than walking. The UK is not particularly cycle-friendly, although it's getting better, and the number and extent of cycle paths is increasing. Too often though they are an after-thought, sharing a narrow strip of the edge of the road with heavy traffic. This contrasts with countries like the Netherlands where cycle paths are the rule rather than the exception. However, cycling is rapidly gaining in popularity and the recent British successes at the Olympics and the Tour de France, as well as cycle-hire schemes in cities such as London, are adding to a real shift in the adoption of cycling both as a leisure activity and transport alternative. Some workplaces are becoming more cycle friendly, offering changing and showering facilities as well as secure cycle-parking areas. Like walking, cycling to work or to the shops provides excellent exercise.

Once you have got your cycling technique working smoothly – if you are new to cycling, make sure you have your bike properly fitted and have someone who is knowledgeable about cycling explain a bit about braking, how to use the right gears, smooth pedal action and the importance of getting your bike serviced annually. Then you are all set for a sport for life. And, of course, you can share the fun of it with family and friends of all ages. When you and your bike are working perfectly and you can hear the machinery singing along, you will get a natural high; you don't have to be a world-class athlete to achieve this, but you can certainly feel like one. And as you start to get more fit and increase your endurance, you may want to try mountain biking. Out on the trails on a summer afternoon with the smell of pine and granite in the air – it doesn't get any better than that!

If your work is further away, consider whether it is possible to use public transport. And if there isn't a bus stop right outside your home or work, so much the better as the walk at either end will do you good! And if there is a bus stop right outside your work, get off at the stop before to increase the walking distance. Okay, you need to get to the office promptly, but it's your long-term health we're talking about here. Do you take children to school by car? Walking with them will not only help your health: it will benefit theirs too.

If you have to use the car to do the weekly shop, increase the distance you have to walk by parking as far away from the shop entrance as you can – where you can usually find lots of free spaces in any case.

Sell your car. Forty years ago, it was almost unheard of for families to have more than one car; somehow they managed to survive. If a couple shares one car, only one of them can drive it at any one time, which means the other one will have to manage without it. As long as it is shared fairly, both will necessarily have to engage in more active travel, by walking, cycling or using public transport.

Get a dog. Dogs need walks and they need their owners to take them. A recent survey revealed that 25 per cent of non-pet owners said they never exercised, compared with 12 per cent of dog owners. Taking a dog out for a walk in the evening will not only increase your activity time, it will also reduce your sedentary time.

If your job involves long periods of sitting, try and get up for a couple of minutes every hour to break your sedentary time. Are there any tasks you can do standing rather than sitting? Is there scope to change your job to one that involves more physical activity?

Consider cutting down the time spent watching television. Remember that just two hours a day of television increases the risk of diabetes by 20 per cent. Given that diabetes is reversible, reducing television time should be seen as part of your strategy to reverse your diabetes. You could set yourself a target of having one or two television-free days each week, or only watching television between certain times. And the same applies to computer time, especially if you play hours of computer games. If you find it difficult to cut down television time, try to get up and move around between each programme, and try to avoid eating while watching the box.

Get a hobby. Learn to play a musical instrument. If you have read this far, it must be obvious by now that activities that involve using and moving muscles are what really matter. Playing the piano consumes calories; playing the saxophone consumes even more. Both involve movement and the use of various muscles. Both will get you away from the television or computer, and should even be enjoyable for you (and those who listen to you, possibly).

Join a club. Preferably one that doesn't involve eating or drinking too much. It doesn't have to be a sports club (although well-managed cycling, running, tennis, sailing clubs, etc., will always supply you with a 'training' routine, discipline and extra motivation when you need it). Try anything that will get you involved in an activity and it's even better if you can walk or cycle there.

Finally, there is increasing evidence that short bursts of high intensity training (HIT for short) can be very effective at burning off fat. This does require the ability to be able to run or cycle (or use an exercise bike) at very high intensity, preferable three times a week. However, the good news is that just 20 seconds' high intensity exercise, repeated after a few minutes of gentle exercise (so that's 40 seconds in total) is enough to make a difference. Dr Michael Mosley's book on the subject, *Fast Exercise*, provides a very interesting account of HIT and a number of examples of how to put it into practice.[13]

In summary, any way in which you are able to increase your physical activity and reduce the time sitting down will help reverse your diabetes. Towards the end of the book we will consider how you can set your own goals to help reverse your diabetes. So have a think about one change that you can make that will get you walking more and sitting less.

CHAPTER 13

APPROPRIATE BLOOD GLUCOSE MONITORING

Our aim in managing type 2 diabetes is to achieve blood glucose values that are as near to normal as possible. In someone with normal glucose metabolism this will generally mean a value of no more than 5.5mmol/l while fasting (such as first thing in the morning) and before meals, and no more than 7.8mmol/l after meals. This chapter will address how you can monitor your progress in reversing your diabetes and make sure you are on track to achieve your goals.

Until the late 1980s, the only method available for a person with diabetes to monitor their diabetic control was by checking the level of glucose in the urine. This involved peeing some urine into a container and dipping a plastic strip with chemicals embedded at one end into the urine. The chemicals reacted with the glucose in the urine, causing the colour of the strip to change according to the amount of glucose in the urine. The colour was then compared with a colour chart to give an indication of how much glucose was present in the urine. Such strips are still available and similar strips are also available to check the level of protein and ketones (see chapter 2) and many other constituents in the urine.

Before the development of strips in the 1970s, checking the glucose in the urine involved peeing into a container, then adding tablets containing the chemicals and observing the colour change and before this the technique involved boiling the urine! Urine test strips are therefore a huge advance on what was previously available. They are cheap and easy to use and, as a result, many people with type 2 diabetes are encouraged to use the method to monitor their diabetes. However, in my view they are a waste of time for the following reasons:

1. Urine testing relies on the kidneys excreting glucose from the urine when levels in the blood rise too high. However, glucose generally does not appear in the urine until the level in the blood is over 10mmol/l, which is much too high for anyone aiming for good control of his or her diabetes. In some people, especially in the elderly, glucose levels can rise even higher before appearing in the urine.

2. Urine is constantly formed by the kidneys and then passes into the bladder where it is stored until a person next urinates, which could be several hours later. Consequently, a urine test is always 'out of date' and does not reflect the level of glucose in the blood at the time the urine is tested.

3. Anyone taking the new SGLT2 class of drugs will have excess glucose in their urine (this is how it works), and so the amount of glucose in the urine will no longer reflect the level in the bloodstream.

4. Urine testing, by definition, means that you have to have some urine in your bladder to pee, and that you can find a loo.

The one situation where urine testing can be helpful is when people are first diagnosed with type 2 diabetes, when they will often (but not always) have glucose in their urine. As they make changes to their diet the amount of glucose in the urine will gradually reduce and after a few weeks, if all goes well, will disappear altogether. Seeing this process in action by testing can be encouraging in that it shows that the lifestyle changes made are having the desired effect – as less glucose in the urine means the blood glucose level is falling. However, once the urine tests are always negative, urine testing is no longer any use in helping monitor blood glucose levels. To do this reliably requires the use of home blood glucose testing.

As urine test strips were developed, similar technology was used to develop strips that measured the level of glucose in the blood. The earliest strips changed colour according to the blood glucose level, and were read in the same way as urine test strips. By the late 1980s meters became available that read the colour change automatically and gave a digital read-out of the result. However, the testing routine was still quite cumbersome: first a person had to prick their finger and squeeze a drop of blood on to the end of the strip; they then had to wait exactly 60 seconds before wiping the blood off the strip, and then wait another 60 seconds to read the colour of the strip. Nowadays many meters produce an accurate blood result in about five seconds.

Blood testing has the obvious disadvantage that you need to prick your finger to get some blood out. If you do lots of tests this can make your fingers quite sore. It can also be quite inconvenient, especially for people who work in dirty environments or who handle food or who are not easily able to wash their hands (which is a requirement for an accurate result). Despite these drawbacks blood testing provides an accurate record of the blood glucose level at the precise time the test is done. This means it can be very useful, not only in checking the fasting glucose level, but also in seeing what effect eating a meal has on the glucose level. For anyone who wishes to monitor his or her diabetes control on a regular basis then blood testing is the only option.

Over the past 10 years there has been a lot of controversy about the usefulness of blood testing in people with type 2 diabetes. It is recognised that it is essential for anyone who is on insulin, but apart from that it is not often recommended. Indeed in some areas of the United Kingdom, GPs will not prescribe blood test strips to people with type 2 diabetes. This bias against blood testing has been fuelled by the fact that test strips are relatively expensive (about 30p each) and that they do not often seem to help improve diabetes control. Indeed, there was a study performed in Northern Ireland a few years ago that suggested that doing regular blood tests was associated with increased depression in people with type 2 diabetes who were being treated with diet or tablets.[1]

However, since then a number of other studies have been published that suggest that using blood tests can have positive effects on both diabetes control and well-being. The key here is not just blood testing but structured testing. By that I mean testing in a structured manner in order to provide specific information that can be useful not only in monitoring a person's diabetes, but also in providing specific feedback – which can be very encouraging when the tests suggest that things are moving in the right direction. There are three types of structured testing I would recommend.

The first is to check the fasting blood glucose on a representative day once a week (e.g. every Wednesday). This is what I call maintenance testing for people whose diabetes is already well controlled. It can also be used alongside the second type of testing described below. As long as the test is within the desired range (usually 4–6mmol/l) and the HbA1c is within range or coming down towards the target, then no further tests need be done. If on a particular week the fasting level is raised, then the test can be repeated for the next two days. If all three tests are high, then more intensive testing may be necessary as described below. My team undertook some preliminary evaluation of this routine some years ago and found it was effective in helping people maintain stable control of their diabetes.[2]

The second type of structured testing is paired mealtime testing. This is where someone checks his or her blood glucose just before a meal and then two hours later. Ideally the glucose level should stay about the same, or rise by at most 2–3mmol/l. Using such results, a person can learn to adjust their diet using the principles described in earlier chapters, until the post-meal test falls within the desired range. This means that the amount of carbohydrate in that particular meal is within a range that the individual is capable of dealing with (assisted by any medications they are taking). If a particular meal leads to a big rise in blood glucose after two hours, then the person can reduce the amount of carbohydrate in it next time they eat that meal. Performing a paired test for one meal once or twice a week has been shown to help people achieve better control of their diabetes.[3] And once a person has identified that they can eat a particular portion (say of rice) without adversely affecting their glucose control, they no longer need to test whenever they eat the same portion of rice.

The third type of structured testing is a seven-point profile. This involves doing a blood test before and after the three main meals of the day and also at bedtime. This should be done if an individual's weekly fasting tests are getting higher in order to determine whether any additional dietary changes ought to be made. It has also been shown that performing a seven-point profile for three consecutive days once every three months can help people with type 2 diabetes, treated with diet or tablets, to achieve better overall control of their diabetes.[4] It would appear that just doing the tests has an effect on his or her behaviour, and often the results are lower for the third day than the first. This is probably because someone seeing high values on the first day makes changes to their diet – consciously or not. This particular type of testing has not only been shown to help people achieve better control of their diabetes, but to increase their well-being. This is in contrast to studies of unstructured testing, and is likely to be a result of the fact that a structured approach enables the person to make changes that lead to better glucose control.

If you are newly diagnosed with type 2 diabetes then I would recommend the once-a-week maintenance test for the first four weeks or so, as this is sufficient to show glucose levels falling as dietary changes are made. Once the fasting level is below 10mmol/l, then paired testing can be introduced, for example for two different meals a week, to enable you to learn the effect of different meals on your glucose control. A three-day seven-point profile (as described above) could then be performed after three months to help you and your doctor assess your overall progress. Once glucose levels are approaching the normal range, a long-term testing strategy might include a fasting test every two weeks, occasional paired mealtime tests (say once a week) and a three-day seven-point profile every three months. Using this programme, a pot of 50 test strips should last about three months.

Home blood testing is not regarded as essential for the management of type 2 diabetes, unless treated with insulin. However, without testing, it is not possible to know how effective lifestyle changes are in achieving stable blood glucose levels. I do therefore recommend testing as described in this chapter so that the effects of changes to diet can be monitored, and to provide much needed encouragement once you see that the changes are working. As I mentioned earlier in this chapter, the use of blood glucose testing in type 2 diabetes is a controversial topic, and not all GPs will be willing (or allowed) to prescribe test strips. In this situation some people are happy to buy their own test strips, which, if used sparingly, would work out at less than £8 per month.

The aim of home glucose monitoring is to guide day-to-day decisions about food intake and activity levels. Long-term monitoring is done by having an HbA1c check every three to six months. As mentioned in chapter 2, an

HbA1c of less than 53mmol/mol (7 per cent) represents good control of diabetes. Reversal of diabetes requires a level of less than 42mmol/mol (6 per cent), through lifestyle changes. Trying to achieve such low levels with medications, especially sulfonylureas and insulin, can be harmful, and is not recommended. Medication certainly has an important role in controlling type 2 diabetes, especially in those for whom reversal may not be feasible. Medications that encourage weight loss can also help towards reversal of diabetes, as we will now discuss in the next chapter.

CHAPTER 14

THE APPROPRIATE USE
OF MEDICATION

In chapter 4 we learnt about the traditional medical treatments for diabetes – tablets such as metformin and sulfonylureas and insulin injections. These were the mainstay of treatment for type 2 diabetes until the early part of the 21st century, and were often prescribed without much attention being paid to lifestyle changes or to supporting patients who wished to make the changes. It was generally accepted that type 2 diabetes was an irreversible, progressive condition and that over time everyone would eventually end up on insulin. Depending on his or her outlook this could well lead to an encroaching sense of pessimism and a feeling that there was no point in trying to make changes to diet and lifestyle if it wasn't going to make much difference in the end. As a result, doctors' training focused almost exclusively on the use of medications to control diabetes; as these medications were limited, insulin ended up being used with increased frequency, especially after the publication in 1998 of the United Kingdom Prospective Diabetes Study (UKPDS) that showed that reducing glucose levels was associated with reduced frequency of complications of diabetes, particularly eye disease. Interestingly, it also showed that, if anything, reducing blood pressure was even more important as this led to reductions in the risk of heart attack and stroke disease.

As discussed in chapter 5, there is now plenty of evidence that obesity is a major risk factor for type 2 diabetes. There has been a marked increase in obesity rates over recent years: in 1993, 13 per cent of men and 16 per cent of women were obese; in 2011, this rose to 24 per cent for men and 26 per cent for women. Current trends suggest that by 2025, 47 per cent of men and 36 per cent of women will be obese.[1] During 2011/12 there were 11,736 hospital admissions due to obesity; incredibly, this was over 11 times higher than during 2001/02.

Against this background, while reducing blood glucose levels will help reduce some of the small vessel diseases associated with diabetes, using insulin to achieve this no longer seems like such a good idea. As we have seen, the problem in type 2 diabetes is that the body cannot use insulin very well. So just giving more insulin is rather missing the point. Insulin itself leads to weight gain; giving it to a population that is already overweight really isn't a good strategy. But for many years that is all we had at our disposal.

Until the 1990s, when a person was already on metformin and a sulfonylurea but still finding that his or her diabetes was not well controlled, the usual practice was to stop the tablets and to start insulin. Doctors then realised that if metformin was continued after insulin was started the metformin seemed to make the insulin work better, and patients would require a lower dose of insulin to achieve good control of their diabetes. This in turn meant they were at less risk of gaining weight. This was the beginning of a trend to move away from concentrating merely on glucose levels, but also taking into account the negative effects of insulin, and the need to minimise the amount of insulin needed, if at all possible. This observation has helped lead to the recognition that metformin is a very effective drug in the treatment of type 2 diabetes.

GLITAZONES

This change in focus led to the search for medications to help the body make better use of insulin – that is to reduce insulin resistance. The first of these was a drug called troglitazone, which was introduced with great fanfare in 1997. It was the first of a new type of drug known as the thiazolidinediones (TZDs or glitazones for short). They work by activating genes in the tissues, especially in the liver, muscle and fat, that increase the sensitivity of the insulin receptors on cells so that more glucose is taken up by the cells after meals; they also seem to cause less glucose to be released from the liver into the bloodstream. The net result is lower glucose levels in the blood. Unfortunately, it soon became apparent that serious liver disease was developing in a small number of patients who took troglitazone. The drug was withdrawn from the UK market after just a few months.

A few years later rosiglitazone was introduced. This did not appear to have any adverse effects on the liver, but even before it was launched there were questions about its safety as there was some evidence in trials that it was associated with increased cholesterol levels and heart problems. However, the manufacturers were able to reassure the regulatory authorities that it was safe, and it was launched in the UK in 1999. I recall the excitement at the time: by treating insulin resistance with rosiglitazone we would get to the heart of the problem in type 2 diabetes, and revolutionise its treatment. For a while all seemed to go well – rosiglitazone did lead to reductions in glucose levels meaning less people needed to start on insulin. Bizarrely, however, many patients gained weight – sometimes quite a lot of it. And as a result, over time, the drug's effectiveness would reduce. Reports also began to emerge of patients developing heart problems. After a number of studies suggested that rosiglitazone was indeed bad for the heart, it was withdrawn from the UK in 2010.[2]

The third glitazone was pioglitazone. This appeared to be safer for the heart and once rosiglitazone was withdrawn, many patients were switched to it. However, reports have subsequently emerged of a link between it and bladder cancer[3] and pioglitazone has now been withdrawn in France and Germany – although it is still available in the UK. Both pioglitazone and rosiglitazone have also been linked to an increased risk of fractures.[4]

As a result, today pioglitazone is rarely recommended as a treatment for type 2 diabetes. If you are taking pioglitazone, and your diabetes is well controlled, then it may be that the benefits outweigh any potential risks. However, if your diabetes is not well controlled, you may wish to consider stopping it. If you go ahead and adopt some of the lifestyle recommendations in this book you may not need to replace it with another drug.

THE GILA MONSTER:
GLP-1 ANALOGUES

Just as the glitazones were fading away, the new kids arriving on the block were the GLP-analogues. The first was Byetta (exenatide), which was introduced in the UK in 2007, followed in 2009 by Victoza (liraglutide) and in 2013 by Lyxumia (lixisenatide).

These drugs are based on a substance called exendin-4 that is found in the saliva of the Gila monster (*Heloderma suspectum*), a venomous lizard found in the south-west United States and in north Mexico. Exendin-4 has similar actions to the human hormone glucagon-like peptide 1 (or GLP-1) that is produced in the gut after a meal, and has a number of beneficial effects:

- It increases the release of insulin from the pancreas
- It suppresses the release of glucagon (glucagon, also released by the pancreas, is the hormone that increases blood glucose levels)
- It slows down the rate at which food leaves the stomach and enters the small intestine. This reduces the speed at which glucose is absorbed into the bloodstream
- It has an effect in reducing appetite, and thereby promotes weight loss

Byetta is a synthetic form of exendin-4 that is given by injection twice daily. As a result of the above effects it leads to lower glucose levels and, sometimes, to quite significant weight loss. It has also been shown to reduce the amount of fat in the liver, probably as a result of weight loss. However, Byetta is also associated with side effects, most noticeably a feeling of nausea leading to loss of appetite. In a sense this is how it works – by significantly reducing the appetite, people eat less. However, in some people the nausea is very troublesome and in certain cases can be associated with vomiting. In such instances, the drug has to be stopped.

Byetta has also been associated with inflammation of the pancreas (pancreatitis),[5] which can be a very serious condition. It is not known quite why this association is present, or even whether it is the Byetta that is the culprit, but as a precaution it cannot be used in anyone who has had pancreatitis in the past.

Victoza and Lyxumia are similar products but only need to be given once a day. Side effects are less marked, so extreme nausea is less of a problem, although it does sometimes occur. They also cannot be used in anyone with a history of pancreatitis. More recently, a long-acting version of Byetta has been launched, called Bydureon. This only needs to be given once a week and may be suitable for people who are unable to inject themselves every day.

Although these drugs do increase insulin levels, their distinct advantage is that they only increase insulin levels after a meal, unlike treatments such as sulfonylureas or insulin injections that increase insulin levels for several hours, regardless of whether a meal has been eaten or not. This can result in excess insulin in the bloodstream when it is not needed, and that will lead to abnormally low blood glucose levels, or hypoglycaemia. With GLP-1 analogues, there is much less risk of hypoglycaemia.

These new drugs generated a lot of excitement when they first appeared, and unlike many other diabetes treatments they led to improved glucose control *and* weight loss. However, over time, the initial excitement is starting to wane. It appears these drugs are not particularly effective in people with very high glucose levels, and in such cases insulin may be required, even if only temporarily. In addition, I have seen many patients who initially had a very good response to Byetta and Victoza, with improved HbA1c levels and weight loss, but after a couple of years their HbA1c, and sometimes their weight, began to rise again. People taking these drugs can develop antibodies to them, and in the case of Byetta, some who have antibodies seem to have a reduced response to the drug. Theoretically, one can imagine that if a person has antibodies to the drug, they will bind to the drug molecules in the bloodstream and neutralise the drug's effect. Whether this is the cause or not, these drugs have not lived up to their initial promise.

In my experience they are most effective in people who have also made significant changes to their diet, and, as discussed in chapter 9, some studies have shown that when combined with a low-calorie diet, these drugs can be very effective in helping people lose a significant amount of weight.

THE GLIPTINS

Naturally occurring GLP-1 is rapidly broken down in the body by an enzyme called Dipeptidyl peptidase-4 (DPP4). The gliptins are a class of drugs that was launched about the same time as the GLP-1 analogues. They act by blocking the action of DPP4, so that the natural GLP-1 lasts longer. The advantage over the GLP-1 drugs is that gliptins can be taken by tablet. While they can sometimes be quite effective, they are not as powerful as the GLP-1 analogues, and again, in some people the effect may not last more than a couple of years. Like the GLP-1 analogues they cannot be used in people who have a history of pancreatitis. One advantage of the gliptins is that some of them can be used in people with quite advanced kidney disease. There are currently five drugs in this class, as shown in the table on p. 186.

THE RISK OF PANCREATIC CANCER

During 2013 concerns began to surface that not only are GLP-1 analogues and gliptins potentially associated with an increased risk of pancreatitis, they might also lead to the development of pancreatic cancer. This concern arose from experiments in rats, where the animals given the drugs developed changes in their pancreases that might lead to cancer. It is important to note that no increase in cases of pancreatic cancer have been observed in the many thousands of people taking these drugs, and I am not aware of any patients in whom pancreatic cancer has occurred. However, it does highlight the importance of being very careful about what drugs you take, and that you understand the potential risk of side effects as well as the benefits.

OTHER DIABETES DRUGS

The meglitinides are a group of drugs that are similar to sulfonylureas in that they act to increase insulin secretion from the pancreas. They are, however, quite short acting, which makes them ideal to be taken with meals and with a theoretical lower risk of hypoglycaemia when compared with longer-acting drugs. In practice they are not noticeably better than short-acting sulfonylureas such as tolbutamide (which is much cheaper). There are two meglitinides – repaglinide and nateglinide as shown in the table.

Acarbose was launched in Germany in 1990 and in the UK a few years later. It works by blocking the breakdown of starches into glucose in the gut. This reduces the absorption of glucose into the bloodstream and can be very effective in lowering blood glucose levels. However, it does have one rather major drawback: as starch is not broken down as normal in the gut, the starch finds itself lower down the gut where it is not normally meant to be found. Here bacteria, which usually reside in the gut, ferment it – producing copious amounts of gas. This can cause bloating, discomfort and a lot of flatulence. These side effects were too embarrassing for many people in the UK and it never really took off. For many years it was the top-selling diabetes drug in Germany. I am really not sure if this was because, somehow, the starch in the German diet acted differently to that in the UK, or whether Germans were simply less bothered about the side effects. Either way, it provides an interesting example of how, even within Europe, cultural differences can have a significant influence on whether a treatment is acceptable or not. Acarbose is still available in the UK and some patients continue to take it. However, I am inclined to think that reducing the amount of carbohydrates eaten is likely to be a more acceptable way of achieving the same result.

SGLT2 INHIBITORS

The most recent addition to the diabetes drugs cupboard is a group of drugs known as SGLT2 inhibitors. In chapter 3 we learnt that the kidneys act as a filter to keep the correct balance in the blood of a number of substances, one of which is glucose. So if glucose levels rise too high, the excess glucose is filtered out through the kidneys. This leads to increased water loss through the kidneys, marked by increased urination, dehydration and excessive thirst. Glucose in the urine is also associated with frequent urinary infections. Until recently these were seen as bad signs, signs that diabetes was not well controlled.

Now this is all set to change as a new class of drugs influences the kidneys' function to make them excrete more glucose in order to reduce the amount of glucose in the bloodstream. There is some interesting evidence that these drugs are associated with an increase in insulin sensitivity, possibly as a result of lower glucose in the bloodstream. However, rather surprisingly, they may also lead to more glucose being released into the bloodstream through an increased effect of glucagon[6]. The implications

DRUGS AVAILABLE TO TREAT DIABETES (IN 2014)

Class of drug	Drug name	Brand name
Biguanide	Metformin	Glucophage
DPP4 inhibitor ('Gliptin')	Alogliptin	Nesina
	Linagliptin	Trajenta
	Saxagliptin	Onglyza
	Sitagliptin	Januvia
	Vildagliptin	Galvus
GLP1-analogue	Exenetide	Byetta Bydureon
	Liraglutide	Victoza
	Lixisenatide	Lyxumia
Meglitinide	Nateglinide	Starlix
	Repaglinide	Prandin
Sulfonylurea	Glibenclamide	Daonil
	Glimepiride	Amaryl
	Gliclazide	Diamicron
	Glipizide	Glucotrol
	Tolbutamide	Orinase
SGLT2 inhibitor	Canagliflozin	Invokana
	Dapagliflozin	Forxiga
Thiazolidinedione ('Glitazone')	Pioglitazone	Actos
Alpha-glucosidase inhibitor	Acarbose	Glucobay

of these effects are not yet known. It is clear, however, that the action of causing excess leakage of calories (in the form of glucose) in the urine, means these drugs may help people with weight loss, and this in turn may help reverse the disease process.

It is important to be aware that increasing the excretion of glucose in the urine risks causing dehydration and urinary infections; indeed these have been reported as side effects. We do not know about the long-term effects of increasing glucose concentration in the urine – which is what will happen when taking these drugs over many years. Finally, using SGLT2 inhibitors will make using urine testing for glucose completely useless as a means of assessing diabetes control.

HOW SHOULD DRUGS BE USED IN TYPE 2 DIABETES?

So what role should drugs play in the management of type 2 diabetes? As we have already discussed, in most cases type 2 diabetes is a disease of our modern-day lifestyle and consequently the most effective treatment is lifestyle change. For some people the lifestyle changes recommended in this book are going to be too difficult, and they will be unable to achieve the weight loss required to control their diabetes. For others, despite their best efforts, his or her glucose levels might remain too high, possibly because there has been irreversible damage to the pancreas. In others, possibly at the time of diagnosis, or during periods of illness, glucose levels may just be too high for lifestyle changes to make much difference. I will cover this scenario first, as the principles of treatment used are very different from the other situations where drugs may be used.

Using medication when glucose levels are very high

When glucose levels are very high (e.g. blood glucose above approximately 15mmol/l or HbA1c above 86mmol/mol or 10 per cent) insulin itself becomes less effective and this can make it very difficult for lifestyle changes to work effectively. At these levels people often experience unpleasant symptoms and feel quite unwell; they are also at greater risk of infections, and it is important to try to bring glucose levels down quite quickly. This situation is seen in some people when they are first diagnosed with type 2 diabetes; it can also be seen in people with established diabetes when they become acutely unwell, for example with a severe infection or when using certain medications such as steroids that act against the effect of insulin and cause elevated glucose levels.

In the case of the newly diagnosed there may be some dietary changes that will make a big difference. For example, if someone has a very high-sugar diet then just eliminating sugar from the diet may in itself bring the blood glucose down to a more manageable level. However, often this is not the case and medication is required. In this situation we need to use medication that will directly reduce glucose levels, and this means using insulin or a sulfonylurea. If the person has lost a lot of weight (which in this situation is not actually a good sign as it means glucose levels have been very high), or if they have been experiencing quite marked symptoms such as extreme thirst, passing large volumes of urine, or blurred vision, then I would generally suggest they start insulin. I would explain that this is a temporary measure (unless I suspect they may in fact have type 1 diabetes – see chapter 2), designed to reduce the blood glucose to a level at which lifestyle changes will be more effective. If his or her symptoms are milder, then I may suggest a sulfonylurea first, such as glipizide. If glucose levels remain raised after a few days then this can be switched to insulin.

The idea of temporary insulin treatment is really quite new; although some people have advocated giving insulin to all patients for a time after the diagnosis of type 2 diabetes to 'rest' the pancreas, this is not feasible in routine clinical practice, and in my view is unnecessary in the majority of cases. In general terms, it was previously felt that if someone needed insulin, they would require it for the rest of their life. My experience of treating people with type 2 diabetes over recent years, and a greater understanding about the reversibility of type 2 diabetes, has taught me that this is definitely not the case.

If insulin is to be started in someone with type 2 diabetes, it is common practice that this is started as a once daily injection of a long-acting insulin such as Humulin I,

Lantus or Levemir. The starting dose can be quite low, as even a small amount of insulin can have a marked effect. The dose can then be gradually increased until fasting glucose levels come down into single figures. Once this happens, the dose can then be reduced again quite rapidly, and often stopped after a few months. As the insulin dose is reduced, metformin can be started, to be continued long-term after the insulin has been stopped. The same approach can be used when a sulfonylurea is used as the initial treatment to reduce glucose levels, whereby the dose is reduced as the glucose levels come down.

The other situation where this approach is used is in patients who develop an acute illness such as an infection. All types of stress, both physical and mental, cause glucose levels to rise, and infection or inflammation cause real stress to the system. It triggers the immune system to rally the body's defences against the illness, and the hormone system to increase levels of adrenaline and cortisol. These so-called 'fight or flight' hormones raise glucose levels to provide energy to fight the illness. When insulin works normally this does not cause a problem; however, in people with diabetes this can cause the blood glucose to rise to a very high level as the body cannot produce extra insulin to push glucose into the muscles and other tissues where it is needed. It is not uncommon to find that someone who has good control of their diabetes, when they are well, may experience high glucose levels when they become ill. This may require insulin, which can be stopped once they have recovered from the illness.

Managing this situation will be described in more detail in the next chapter.

The final situation, where insulin or sulfonylureas are used, is when other treatments designed to reduce insulin resistance do not lead to the required level of glucose control. In this situation the treatment does become long term, and one may have to accept the risks of increasing insulin levels still further, such as causing increased weight gain as the cost of achieving the benefits of good glucose control.

Using medication following diagnosis

At diagnosis, unless glucose levels are very raised – in which case insulin or a sulfonylurea may be advised – the general advice is to try and maximise insulin sensitivity (or reduce insulin resistance). Initially, this will involve encouraging the person to make changes to their lifestyle, predominantly their diet. If, after three months, glucose levels are still elevated (i.e. fasting glucose is above 7mmol/l) then medication may be considered. In most cases this will involve the prescription of metformin, which, as discussed in chapter 4, works by increasing insulin sensitivity. As metformin does not lead to weight gain, and in general is very safe, then its use is consistent with the general principles recommended in this book, namely to enhance the sensitivity of insulin and thereby make it easier to lose weight. As also discussed in chapter 4, metformin can be associated with unpleasant side effects, and in order to minimise them it is generally suggested metformin is started at a low dose, such as 500mg once a day before a meal. After a week, the dose can then be increased to one tablet twice a day. After another week, the dose can be increased to two tablets in the morning and one in the evening, and then after another week, to the maximum dose of two tablets twice a day. However, if despite a low dose metformin cannot be tolerated then an alternative option would be a gliptin, such as sitagliptin or saxagliptin, as first-line treatment.

If despite first-line treatment, glucose levels remain elevated, then another type of drug can be added. If metformin is the first line drug, it makes sense to add a gliptin as second-line if the person is moderately overweight (BMI less than 30), or to add a GLP-1 analogue such as Byetta or Victoza if they are obese (BMI over 30). However, I think it is essential to use this opportunity not just to prescribe another drug, but to review what lifestyle changes he or she has made, and discuss what further changes might be possible, in order to maximise the effectiveness of the drug. In all honesty, if a person is still eating 4,000 calories a day and consuming large amounts of carbohydrate-rich food, then there seems little point in adding more medications which are unlikely to make much difference.

If a gliptin was the first-line drug, then this can be switched to a GLP-1 analogue in those who are obese; in those who are not obese the choice becomes more limited. As discussed in chapter 4, pioglitazone is probably not ideal as it can cause weight gain (and other complications). It may be that an SGLT2 inhibitor will be helpful at this stage. Acarbose may be worth a try, but if not then a sulfonylurea or insulin is the next step. If either of these is to be introduced, my general approach would be to suggest adding these to the current treatment. Remember that while insulin and sulfonylureas can in many cases lead to good control of diabetes, they increase insulin levels and are therefore unlikely to lead to reversal of the diabetes disease process.

In summary, drug treatment of type 2 diabetes can be very useful in the short term when glucose levels are very high. In all other situations, metformin, gliptins and GLP-1 analogues are the only drugs that are likely to help with the process of reversing diabetes. SGLT2 inhibitors are still quite new, but these may have a beneficial effect. It is important that any drug should be seen as supporting changes to diet and lifestyle rather than curative treatments in themselves. Given concerns about their safety, treatment with gliptins and GLP-1 analogues should be reviewed on a regular basis. Where lifestyle changes cannot be made or do not lead to significant control of glucose levels, then long-term treatment with a sulfonylurea or insulin may be required. These recommendations are summarised in the table overleaf.

SUGGESTED APPROACHES TO THE USE OF MEDICATION IN TYPE 2 DIABETES

Treatment stage	Drug class	Examples of drug and dose	Notes
1	Lifestyle change		
2	Metformin	Start 500mg once daily, increase gradually to 1g twice daily	If unable to tolerate, try slow-release preparation and/or move to stage 3. Stop during severe illness or if GFR < 30§
3a (If BMI <30, or in BMI>30 if unwilling to use injections) OR	Gliptin	Saxagliptin 5mg* Sitagliptin 100mg**	Add to metformin *2.5mg if GFR <30 **25mg if GFR <30
3b (If BMI > 30) OR	GLP1 analogue	Exenatide (Byetta) 5mcg twice daily, increasing to 10mcg after 4 weeks Liraglutide (Victoza) 0.6mg once daily increasing to 1.2mg after 2 weeks	Add to metformin

Treatment stage	Drug class	Examples of drug and dose	Notes
3c (if gliptin or GLP1 analogue not suitable or tolerated)	SGLT2 inhibitor	Canagliflozin 100mg, increasing to 300mg once daily Dapagliflozin 10mg daily	Add to metformin
4a (If HbA1c <80 or unwilling to take injections) OR	Sulfonylurea	Glipizide 5mg once daily increasing if necessary to 10mg twice daily. Gliclazide 80mg, increasing to 160mg twice daily	Add to metformin, consider stopping other treatments if no evidence of benefit
4b (If HbA1c >80 or if sulfonylurea ineffective)	Basal insulin	Humulin I, Lantus or Levemir, 10 units once daily, increasing according to blood glucose response	Add to metformin; consider stopping other treatments if no evidence of benefit
5	Mealtime insulin	Humalog or Novorapid, 1-3u per 10g carbohydrate in meals	

§GFR = glomerular filtration rate, a measure of kidney function, assessed by a blood test. The value roughly equates to the percentage of kidney function remaining.

Treatment should progress from stage 1 to 5 in a stepwise fashion as described in the text.

CHAPTER 15

MANAGING WHEN OTHER ILLNESSES STRIKE

It is an unfortunate fact that people with type 2 diabetes are likely to experience other health problems, and when they do, they are likely to be affected more seriously and for longer than people without diabetes. To a large extent this is because type 2 diabetes is itself associated with vascular problems such as coronary artery disease and strokes. However, as has already been discussed, the risks of these can be significantly reduced by ensuring good control of blood pressure and cholesterol levels. Taking steps to reverse your diabetes by losing weight and adjusting your diet is likely to further reduce this level of risk, although it is too early for this to have been proven by clinical trials.

The other thing that affects how illness affects a person with type 2 diabetes is the level of glucose in the bloodstream. A high blood glucose level affects the body's functioning in two important ways: it can lead to dehydration and low blood pressure, which may adversely affect kidney function; it can also make one more susceptible to infection, and to be affected by the infection more seriously than someone who does not have diabetes. This results from the rather complex effects diabetes can have on the way the body fights infection, and because it is the simple fact that glucose is a fuel for all living organisms – including bacteria that are more likely to thrive in a high-glucose environment. As everyone with diabetes will have glucose levels higher than someone without the disease, just having diabetes increases susceptibility to infection. People whose glucose levels are high will experience more frequent infections, even if they are otherwise well. As excess glucose is excreted in the urine, both bladder infections and thrush are common in people with high levels of glucose in their bloodstream.

The real issues arise in people with problems such as foot ulcers, where infection can very easily get into the local tissues and can be very difficult to treat, especially if the blood supply is diminished by large blood vessel disease. In such situations it is very important to maintain blood glucose levels as near normal as possible, in order to help combat the infection and to stop it from spreading.

The additional risk of infection underlines the importance of maintaining good hygiene and of paying particular attention to the feet. This is particularly important if you have any degree of diabetic nerve disease that causes loss of sensation. If sensation is impaired, you will not be so aware of any cut or graze on your foot and, as a result, such a cut may be left open, providing easy access for bacteria to enter the tissues under the skin. If you have any loss of sensation in your feet it is vital that you, or someone else, checks the skin on your feet, including the soles of your feet, every day, to make sure there are no cuts or scratches. It is also very important not to wear shoes that are too tight, as excess pressure on the skin can cause a blister, which can then break down, causing an ulcer. At the risk of repeating myself: if you have impaired sensation in the feet you might fall into the trap of buying shoes that are too tight as you cannot properly assess the pressure of the shoes on your feet. It is really important that when you buy new shoes you make sure that you are buying the correct size.

As we have already discussed, keeping blood glucose levels as normal as possible will help prevent further health problems, such as eye, foot or kidney disease. It will also help ensure that if you become ill any effect of having diabetes will be minimised. However, it is important to recognise that any illness is a stress on the body, and is associated with increased levels of stress hormones such as cortisol and adrenaline. These hormones counter the effect of insulin, causing glucose to be released from the liver into the bloodstream. Even if your diabetes is generally under very good control, any illness can cause your blood glucose level to rise. While it is true that experiencing high glucose levels for a few weeks (or even months) is unlikely to lead to significant long-term damage, it may mean that the illness takes longer to resolve itself, especially if it involves an infection.

So, it may be necessary to increase diabetes medication in order to control glucose levels during a period of illness. This could mean increasing the dose of tablets or insulin or starting a new tablet or insulin injections for the period of illness. If you are admitted to hospital, your diabetes should be monitored closely and be reviewed by a member of the diabetes team, who will be able to adjust your medication in order to stabilise your diabetes control if it becomes necessary. Very often you will be able to return to your previous treatment before, or shortly after, going home again.

Illness can also cause problems with kidney function, especially in people who have a degree of diabetic kidney disease. We have already mentioned that metformin, which is probably the safest and most effective medication for type 2 diabetes, should not be used in people whose kidney function is impaired. As a rule, anyone who takes metformin should stop taking it if they need to be admitted to hospital with an acute illness, or if they have any illness that causes dehydration, such as prolonged vomiting or diarrhoea, as these are situations that can affect kidney function. If you have impaired kidney function and take medication for high blood pressure, it may be advisable to stop these during periods of illness. It is a good idea to discuss this in advance with your diabetes care team so that you know what to do during periods of illness.

If you manage your diabetes with diet and lifestyle changes alone, it is important to recognise that your glucose levels may be higher than normal during periods of illness. During bouts of illness it is advisable to be particularly careful not to eat or drink sugary foods, and to avoid high-carbohydrate foods. Regular fluids, ideally plain water, should be taken. Even if you do not regularly check your blood glucose, I would suggest checking it at least once a day (perhaps first thing in the morning) when ill. If the level is above 10mmol/l you may need to start taking medication to help control your glucose levels during the period of illness.

If you are on a sulfonylurea or insulin, the dose may need to be increased if glucose levels rise. In some situations, particularly if you are not eating normally, your blood glucose level may fall too low. This is why it is important to check your glucose levels two or three times a day, and if levels are falling below 4mmol/l, the dose of sulfonylurea or insulin will need to be decreased. This is a situation where you should take medical advice on the best course of action.

If you are on a GLP-1 agonist or a gliptin they can usually be continued during illness – unless you have renal disease and become dehydrated. Increasing the dose is unlikely to help control glucose levels, as its effect can take some time. Instead, adding a sulfonylurea or insulin may be required, so if your glucose levels do rise you should seek medical advice.

As previously mentioned, blood pressure medications may need to be stopped if you are experiencing diarrhoea or vomiting which lasts more than a day, especially if you have impaired renal function.

Some medications can also affect glucose control. The most important are steroids, usually taken as tablets such as prednisolone. This is used in high doses for people who have exacerbations of asthma and many other inflammatory conditions. If you need to take steroids, then it is possible you may also need to have insulin (or a higher dose of insulin) while you are on steroids. There are many other tablets that can potentially affect glucose levels. These effects are usually quite mild and we do not have the space to list all of them in this book.[1]

As a general rule I would advise anyone with diabetes who takes medication to discuss with their doctor, in the event of illness, what they should do with each of their medications (both those for diabetes and those for other conditions). In this way you can construct your own 'sick day rules' that should be kept handy, so that you can easily refer to the list if you become unwell. The table opposite provides an example.[1]

Finally, it is important to be aware that even a mild viral illness, which may cause no more than a headache and a runny nose, may have quite a profound effect on blood glucose levels. This is a reflection of your immune system helping your body overcome the infection. It is therefore worthwhile keeping an occasional check on your blood glucose even during mild illnesses.

EXAMPLES OF SICK DAY RULES

Tablet	Dose	Taken for	If I become unwell
Metformin	500mg twice a day	Diabetes	Stop if I have diarrhoea and vomiting
Gliclazide	40mg daily	Diabetes	Check blood sugar levels, may need to increase dose to 80mg (check with doctor)
Ramipril	5mg daily	High blood pressure	Stop if I have diarrhoea and vomiting
Prednisolone	30mg for 5 days	Exacerbation of bronchitis	Increase gliclazide to 80mg twice a day (check with doctor)

So to summarise this chapter: people with diabetes are more likely to become unwell, and when they do this can make their diabetes less well controlled. During any illness it is important to keep track of your glucose levels and to consider adjusting your medication as I have described. This may also apply to someone who, for most of the time, meets the definition of having gone into diabetes remission, that is, someone who has reversed their diabetes and keeps normal glucose levels.

CHAPTER 16

KEEPING BLOOD PRESSURE AND CHOLESTEROL LEVELS UNDER CONTROL

In chapter 3 we discussed the possible complications of diabetes and how high blood pressure and high cholesterol levels contribute to these. It means that it is vital to keep your blood pressure and cholesterol levels as close to normal levels as possible. Having type 2 diabetes means that it is more likely that you will have high blood pressure and higher cholesterol levels than if you do not have the condition. This is at least in part because insulin can, directly or indirectly, affect blood pressure and cholesterol, and insulin resistance is associated with high levels of both.

All this means that if you are able to makes changes to your lifestyle that reduce insulin resistance – reducing insulin and glucose levels in your blood by changing your diet as described in this book – then there is a good chance your cholesterol level and blood pressure will also come down, especially if and when you lose weight. However, as long as your cholesterol and blood pressure remain high, you are at increased risk of developing complications related to large and small blood vessel disease (as described in chapter 3).

HIGH BLOOD PRESSURE

So what exactly is meant by blood pressure? It is exactly what it says it is: the level of pressure that the blood is under in the blood vessels. The cells that make up the body need glucose and oxygen (plus a variety of other substances) to function effectively. The job of blood is to carry these necessary chemicals and nutrients to every part of the body. Blood is also the means by which the hormones produced in the pancreas (such as insulin) are transported to the different parts of the body, where they are needed to perform their biochemical action (in the case of insulin, enabling glucose to enter cells).

So for blood to function effectively it needs nice clean blood vessels to flow through and it needs to be under pressure in order to flow (against the force of gravity a lot of the time). Obviously if there were no pressure the blood would just sit where it is, like a stagnant pool.

Blood pressure comes primarily from the action of the heart, the specialised muscle that acts as a pump squeezing the blood through the arteries. The kidneys also have an important role in controlling blood pressure, both by regulating the amount of water in the blood vessels, and by producing hormones that help control how tight the blood vessels contract (to increase pressure) or relax (to reduce blood pressure). It will be obvious that diseases of either the heart or the kidneys may cause problems with blood pressure regulation – and can make an existing blood pressure problem worse.

So you can see that a vicious circle can develop whereby having type 2 diabetes increases the risk of high blood pressure. This combination in itself can lead to heart and kidney problems and these (especially the kidney problems) can then make the blood pressure problem worse, thus making further complications such as a stroke or heart attack more likely, and so on.

For years, blood pressure was measured by placing an inflatable cuff around the upper arm. The cuff was connected to a machine called a sphygmomanometer, which contained mercury. As the cuff was inflated with a small hand pump, the mercury would rise up a fine glass tube (a bit like a thermometer) as the pressure increased. A doctor or nurse placed a stethoscope over the artery in the arm to listen for the sound of the blood flowing to determine the blood pressure, according to the height of the mercury.

Today blood pressure is measured using a machine connected to the cuff that is still placed tightly around the upper arm. The cuff is inflated until the pressure it exerts around the arm is high enough to stop the blood flowing through the main artery (called the brachial artery, so technically we are measuring arterial blood pressure). The cuff pressure is then gradually decreased until the blood flow returns to normal. As it does, a sensor detects when the cuff reaches the level of the pressure in the arteries as the heart is contracting (called systolic blood pressure) and the level of the pressure as the heart is relaxing (called diastolic blood pressure). These results are then displayed on a digital display as two numbers with the systolic pressure first, for example 120/80. The actual numbers refer to millimetres of mercury (mm Hg), relating back to the days of the original sphygmomanometer.

So what should your blood pressure be? There are many guidelines that specify the ideal levels of blood pressure in different circumstances, but as a general rule it should be below 140/80. If you are young, or have evidence of kidney or eye disease, then a lower level may be recommended. Here it is important to mention that, just like blood glucose, blood pressure levels vary quite considerably during the day, according to what you are doing and experiencing. In fact, blood pressure can rise very quickly if, for example, you get a sudden shock or undertake sudden intense exercise or physical activity. Just as a single blood glucose measurement cannot give an accurate overview of your diabetes control, neither can a single blood pressure measurement be used to determine your blood pressure control.

Ideally, blood pressure should be measured in a relaxed environment after resting for at least five minutes. And yet it is very often measured in a busy clinic setting, perhaps after you have been waiting for some time, getting more and more tense. Some years ago when home blood pressure monitors began to become more widely available, we checked the blood pressure readings of a number of people with diabetes, taken in our clinic, at their GP's surgery, and at home. It came as no surprise to us to find that the highest readings were those taken in the clinic and the lowest readings were taken at home, with those taken in the GP surgery somewhere in between. So if your blood pressure is found to be high at a clinic visit, it is probably worth having it re-checked at your doctor's surgery, or better still, purchase a monitor so that you can check your blood pressure yourself. Again, some years ago we evaluated the accuracy of inexpensive home blood pressure monitors and found them to give similar readings to the much more expensive device we use in our clinics.

I therefore recommend that anyone with diabetes whose blood pressure has been found to be higher than ideal buys a machine for home use. These can be purchased for less than £30. I would suggest checking your blood pressure no more than once every two weeks – just to reassure yourself (and your doctor) that all is well. Obviously if your blood pressure is high, or you are on medication for blood pressure, then more frequent monitoring may be required.

If your blood pressure has been found to be consistently high then you are at increased risk of further health problems, and it is important to try to reduce it. You may well need tablets to achieve this, something we will discuss later. First, however, there may be some lifestyle changes that will help.

Being overweight and inactive is associated with raised blood pressure. So losing weight by modifying your diet and increasing your physical activity (or reducing periods of inactivity), as described in chapter 12, will also have an effect in reducing your blood pressure. However, there are other specific factors that can affect blood pressure: stress, alcohol and salt.

Stress is part of life and for the vast majority of us cannot be avoided. When we are under stress the body produces a number of 'stress hormones' that gear us up for 'fight or flight', which is a deeply instinctive response to either engage in a fight or run away. Part of the actions of these hormones is to increase blood pressure. However, unlike our ancient ancestors, it is very unlikely that the stress we experience will lead either to fight or flight (both of which, incidentally, would use up calories and help keep one fit!) Rather, the hormones adversely affect our blood pressure, and if the stress is frequent or continuous, as is often the case in modern life, then this can lead to long-term problems with high blood pressure – especially in the context of an unhealthy lifestyle with little exercise. So if you recognise that you are under stress, please take time to see what you can do to reduce the stressful elements in your life if at all possible.

Stress sometimes leads to drinking too much alcohol. While there is plenty of evidence to suggest that drinking a moderate amount of alcohol is actually beneficial to health, drinking in excess of the standard guidelines (14 units per week for women, and 21 for men) is associated with a number of health problems, including a rise in blood pressure. So if you drink more than the recommended guidelines – and many of us underestimate the amount of alcohol we drink – then it is likely to be contributing to high blood pressure, and I would recommend you consider how you might cut down. I know of many people who have managed to do this quite successfully by adopting some ground rules for drinking. Examples include: not drinking alcohol alone, not drinking at home, not having beer in the house or nominating two or three days each week when you will not drink alcohol. The important thing is that whatever you decide to do has to be realistic, something that you can keep up – and is not too drastic. Having said that, I know of some people who decided to stop drinking alcohol completely and succeeded in doing so.

The third thing that increases blood pressure is salt. A higher salt level in the body leads to more water remaining in the circulation, which, if excessive, can lead to high blood pressure. Now given that we are largely made up of salty water (or saline), then it is clear that we need some salt in our diet. Indeed, people with too little salt can experience dizziness and fainting owing to their blood pressure being too low. Very low salt concentrations in the blood can cause more severe problems including brain damage. However, our modern diet includes far too much salt. And this is made worse in people with too much insulin, as insulin itself helps the body retain salt, exacerbating the problem. This is one of the reasons why people with insulin resistance and type 2 diabetes have high blood pressure.

If your blood pressure is high, reducing the salt in your diet can make a big difference. The first step is to try to avoid adding salt to your food at the table. Pepper or other spices will add taste with no effect on your blood pressure. Then you should consider reducing the amount of salt you add during cooking. Obviously salt is important to enhance flavour, but not so much that you can actually taste the saltiness. However, the biggest challenge in reducing salt is knowing which foods contain it and in what amounts: something that may surprise you when you get into the detail of it.

Just about any savoury foods (and many sweet foods) that are not fresh will, in all likelihood, have salt added. And this not only includes highly processed foods (such as shop-bought, ready-made meals) that you may well perceive to be unhealthy, but also more traditional foods such as bread, bacon and cheese. Sweet foods, such as breakfast cereals, may also contain salt. Salt is often used to add flavour to low-quality ingredients and, therefore, you may find that cheaper 'value' processed foods have a higher salt content than more expensive ones. In the UK we are fortunate in that many companies have voluntarily reduced the salt content of their foods so we now see lower salt concentrations in many processed foods than will be found in their counterparts in other parts of the world.

If you follow the suggestions in this book then I hope you will eat more fresh foods and less processed food, and this alone will help reduce your intake of salt as well as sugar and fat.

We have already discussed how increasing your activity and reducing periods of inactivity can help you lose weight and improve your diabetes control. The same changes you decide to make, in order to increase your activity level, will over time, also contribute to reducing your blood pressure. If you are significantly overweight, then reducing your body weight will certainly help reduce your blood pressure.

It is possible that despite making changes to your lifestyle and your diet, your blood pressure remains too high – especially if you have had diabetes for some time. In this case, you may need to take medication to reduce your blood pressure.

There are several types of tablets for high blood pressure and those most commonly used for people with diabetes include groups of drugs called ACE inhibitors (or angiotensin-converting-enzyme inhibitors) or ARBs (angiotensin receptor blockers). Examples of these are shown in the table below. Both of these groups of drugs have additional actions in protecting the kidney from the effects of diabetes and are relatively free from side effects. In fact the most common side effect from ACE inhibitors is that they can cause a troublesome dry cough. If that happens, then switching to an ARB usually resolves the problem. Other common blood pressure tablets include mild diuretics (water tablets), calcium-channel blockers, alpha-blockers and beta-blockers. It is not uncommon that a combination of three or more different blood pressure drugs are required in order to achieve good blood pressure control.

Some people may experience different side effects from certain blood pressure tablets, for example, I have known people who feel 'spaced out' on a particular tablet or who experience vomiting. If this happens, it is important to identify which tablet is causing it, and find another that does not cause the problem. One side effect that is quite common is erectile dysfunction, which, as we discussed in chapter 3, can also result from the effects of diabetes. Why should a tablet designed to protect your health make it more difficult to get an erection? The answer lies in the fact that an erection is caused by spaces in the penis called the corpora cavernosa filling up with blood. This requires a good blood flow to be delivered by the arteries supplying the penis. People with high blood pressure are likely to have a degree of narrowing of the arteries (large vessel disease, as discussed in chapter 3), which will reduce the blood flow. Taking a tablet that reduces the blood pressure in the whole circulation is likely to reduce

Class of drug	Examples	Possible side effects	Notes
ACE inhibitor	Ramipril Perindopril Lisinopril	Cough May worsen kidney function	Kidney function should be checked periodically
ARB	Candesartan Irbesartan losartan	May worsen kidney function	Should be stopped during acute illness or dehydration (e.g. diarrhoea and vomiting)
Thiazide diuretic	Bendroflumethazide Chlorthalidone	Low sodium level	
Calcium-channel blocker	Amlodipine Felodipine Nifedipine	Ankle swelling	
Alpha-blocker	Doxasozin	Ankle swelling Dizziness on standing	
Beta-blocker	Bisoprolol Carvedilol Atenolol	Slow pulse	

the blood flow to the penis even more, making it difficult to get an erection. This is why this problem can occur with a variety of different blood pressure medications. Fortunately tablets such as Viagra (they open up the blood spaces in the penis to increase the flow of blood into them) can help.

Earlier in this chapter I mentioned how useful it is to be able to monitor your blood pressure at home, which will help ensure it is under good control. Measuring your blood pressure at home is even more useful if you are on medication. Indeed, I often encourage people to measure their own blood pressure to determine what dose of medication they need. If you are on medication for your blood pressure, I would strongly advise you to purchase a monitor so you can keep a check on it yourself. My general advice is to check your blood pressure once a week, and if it is still too high, to seek advice on how to adjust your medication. You can then take responsibility for making sure your treatment is keeping your blood pressure where it should be.

To summarise: people with diabetes have a tendency to high blood pressure. High blood pressure accelerates some of the complications of diabetes. It is therefore very important that you keep your blood pressure as normal as possible – that is below 140/80. Changing your lifestyle to get more active, to reduce the salt in your diet and to lose weight will all help. Taking medication is often also necessary, and it is very helpful to monitor your blood pressure yourself, to ensure that the treatment is doing what it should be. Finally, you should be aware of the possible side effects of switching to a different treatment.

If your blood pressure is normal, it is really important that it is checked at least once a year, and if it rises above 140/80, that you seek advice on whether treatment is

required. You cannot tell if your blood pressure is high –
the only way of knowing what it is, is to have it checked.

HIGH CHOLESTEROL

The other important risk factor for large vessel disease,
which is the underlying cause of so many problems, is
high cholesterol. Let's be clear: the body needs cholesterol
for many functions. Cell membranes, which control
what enters into cells of the body, are largely made of
cholesterol. Vitamin D, essential for healthy bones,
and many hormones are also made from cholesterol.
However, in today's society, too many of us have too much
cholesterol in our bloodstream, and this predisposes us to
narrowing of the arteries, which can lead to heart attacks,
strokes and gangrene.

There are several types of cholesterol that have different
actions. LDL-cholesterol is made in the liver and released
into the bloodstream where, if too much is produced, it
can cause narrowing of the arteries. HDL-cholesterol, on
the other hand, is good for you.

As a rule, your cholesterol levels should be as follows:

Total cholesterol   less than 5
LDL cholesterol   less than 3
HDL cholesterol   MORE than 1

People who already have evidence of large blood vessel disease, or who are at a high risk of it, are advised to achieve lower targets. Now, some people have a high total cholesterol, but this is because there is a high level of healthy HDL. For this reason it is often easiest to look just at the LDL cholesterol when deciding if you need to make any changes. As with high blood pressure, there are no symptoms associated with having a high cholesterol level, so it is very important to have a blood test done once every year to check your cholesterol level. If your cholesterol levels are higher than they should be then it is important that you know and understand what you can do to reduce them.

As with high blood pressure, the first thing to consider is whether there are any changes you can make to your lifestyle. And the good news is that exactly the same changes that will help reduce your blood pressure will also reduce your cholesterol level. So, increasing your physical activity, eating a healthy diet, and losing weight will all contribute to reducing cholesterol levels. And beware of being taken in by low-fat foods. While there may seem to be a certain logic that says eating less fat will reduce your cholesterol level, remember insulin is the main fat-producing hormone, and reducing your carbohydrate intake (as well as, rather than only, reducing the fat content of meals) will help reduce your insulin level, as well as helping to improve your diabetes control.

There are now a number of foods that have been specially developed that claim to reduce cholesterol levels.

And it's entirely possible they do, but generally only if you take them every day – and that will almost certainly significantly increase your weekly shopping bill. My advice is to eat the natural foods that will help you lose weight, as described in chapter 10. It is also worth remembering that most of the cholesterol in the bloodstream is produced in the liver, and so changing your diet may have only limited effect. The most useful goal is to lose weight, which, as we learned earlier, will reduce the amount of fat found in the liver, and this will in turn help return the liver function to normal, with less production of cholesterol.

Just as with blood pressure, many people with high cholesterol levels may find it necessary to take medication to reduce them. Today, the most common type of medication for high cholesterol levels is a class of drug called statins (such as simvastatin or atorvastatin). Statins all work in a similar way, by reducing the amount of cholesterol released from the liver into the bloodstream. They are undoubtedly effective and are generally well tolerated, and only need to be taken once a day. However, they can cause side effects, particularly when used at higher doses. The most common side effect is the reported incidences of muscle aches and pains. Sometimes this can be associated with a potentially serious inflammation of the muscles known as myositis. However, as statins have become more widely used, a number of other side effects have been reported, ranging from headaches, difficulty in sleeping, joint pains and poor concentration. If you feel that you have experienced a new symptom since taking a statin, my advice would be to stop the statin for a few weeks. Generally, if the symptom is related to the statin, it will soon disappear after stopping the medication. It may be that you will manage better with a lower dose of the statin, or with a different statin. Occasionally alternative types of medication may be required.

If you are unable to tolerate medication you may take some comfort from recent evidence that suggests that adopting a Mediterranean diet is at least as effective in reducing the risk of vascular disease as taking a statin (see note 1, chapter 10). To recap, a Mediterranean diet includes olive oil, legumes, fruits and vegetables, high consumption of fish and low consumption of meat.

High blood pressure and high cholesterol contribute to many of the complications of type 2 diabetes. Keeping them under good control will help reduce the risk of complications. The key steps to achieving this are to know what your own levels are, to improve your diet and to increase your activity levels, and to lose weight (even if you are only marginally overweight).

CHAPTER 17

THE IMPORTANCE OF OTHER HEALTH CHECKS: THE EYES, FEET AND KIDNEYS

THE EYES

In chapter 3 we discussed the different types of complications that can occur if type 2 diabetes is not well controlled, and in the last chapter we talked about the importance of controlling cholesterol and blood pressure levels to minimise the risk of complications. And, in between, we have learned that making lifestyle changes and losing weight can be very effective in reversing some of the processes that contribute to type 2 diabetes. By reducing blood glucose levels, this will also help reduce the risk of complications.

Even if you are doing all these things to reduce the risk of complications, it is still important to have regular health checks performed, usually once a year, to assess whether you have any signs of impending complications that might need treatment. The aim of this chapter is to explain something about each of these checks, and how you should go about getting them done.

Eye checks are important to detect the earliest signs of diabetic eye disease (retinopathy). To recap, the disease usually manifests in the form of abnormalities to small blood vessels. The progress of retinopathy can be halted, and even reversed, by good control of blood glucose and blood pressure. However, the early changes do not affect eyesight and the only way of knowing whether you have them is by having a photograph taken of your retina. In the UK we are fortunate in having a comprehensive eye-screening service, which is free of charge for people with diabetes. This is separate from the usual eye test that you might have to determine if you need glasses.

The test involves drops being put into your eyes that dilate the pupils (making them bigger) so that there is a good view of the retina behind it. You will then be asked to sit still in front of a specialised camera that takes a photograph of your retina through the pupil. The image is usually ready very quickly, and in many cases the person taking it will be able to show it to you. In any case, I would encourage you to ask to see it, as it is your retina after all! Although the operator may be able to give an informal opinion of the image, it will be transmitted to a grading centre, where an expert will assess it for evidence of any diabetic eye disease. In due course, you will receive a letter confirming the findings. If all is well you will be invited back for another test after one or, sometimes, two years. If there is evidence of mild, or background, retinopathy, then you will be advised of this and a further test may be recommended in six or twelve months' time. In the meantime it would be good to consider what you can do to ensure your glucose levels and blood pressure are as well controlled as possible. If the image shows evidence of more severe retinopathy, an appointment will be made for you to see an eye specialist (ophthalmologist) who can perform a more detailed examination and discuss possible treatments with you.

Further information on retinopathy screening can be found at diabeticeye.screening.nhs.uk/diabetic-retinopathy.[1]

Meanwhile the most important thing you can do is to actually turn up for the eye test. Some people have told me how they are fearful of having the test done in case it shows some evidence of diabetic eye disease. While I can understand the quite natural fear, I would urge you not to let it stop you having the test done as – in the early stages – good control of blood glucose levels can stop retinopathy progressing, and even help reverse it. For more advanced disease, treatment is available which can keep it under control and protect your eyesight.

THE FEET

Just as regular eye examinations are important, regular foot examination is a key part of diabetes care. Feet can be affected both by diabetic nerve disease – causing numbness and loss of sensation in your feet – and by blood vessel disease that reduces blood flow. Both of these problems can lead to breakdown of the skin resulting in an ulcer. This in turn can result in infection in the tissues under the skin or in the bone. Poor blood supply can make it difficult to eradicate infection, and can mean the foot has to be amputated.

Throughout this book I have tried to emphasise that a diagnosis of type 2 diabetes no longer means you will inevitably get more and more health problems. However, everyone with the condition must be aware of how diabetes can affect your health, and understand the various strategies to adopt and regular tests to undergo that will combine to keep you healthy. And when it comes to feet, it is important to recognise how quickly problems can occur and how severe they might ultimately prove. I have, for example, seen how quickly people with neuropathy develop foot ulcers as a result of wearing shoes that are too tight. In some cases this has led to deep-seated infection requiring long periods in hospital, and unfortunately in some cases, requiring amputation.

It is a sad fact that once blood vessel disease has set in, it is largely irreversible – especially when it affects the small blood vessels. Although there is evidence that some forms of diabetic nerve disease can improve with good control of diabetes, this may not be enough to avoid problems further down the line. So as far as the feet are concerned, it is important for me to emphasise that it is vital to prevent problems occurring in the first place.

We have already discussed how good control of blood glucose, cholesterol levels and blood pressure can reduce the risk of complications. This is especially important in anyone who already has evidence of blood vessel or nerve disease where a damage limitation exercise is already in play. This is why it is so important that your feet are examined on a regular basis (at least once a year). The examination is relatively straightforward, and includes a check on the pulses in the feet (preferably using a Doppler machine that assesses the flow through the arteries) and a simple check to test sensation. A nylon fibre (called a monofilament) is used to touch the sole of the feet in specific areas to see if you can feel it. The tests may pick up problems before you are aware of them, and if they do, should prompt a review of your diabetes management to ensure that everything is being done to minimise any further damage. Usually the team at your doctor's surgery or at your diabetes clinic carries out these tests, though it does not really matter where the tests are done – the important thing is that they are done and acted upon.

KIDNEY FUNCTION

Kidney function is assessed by means of a blood and a urine test that should be performed once a year. The blood test measures the estimated glomerular filtration rate (or eGFR) and is a measure of kidney function. The eGFR is calculated using a formula that depends on the amount of creatinine in the blood. Creatinine is a by-product of the body's breakdown of protein and is excreted by the kidneys. If the kidneys are not working properly creatinine is not excreted into the urine and, consequently, the amount of creatinine in the blood accumulates. A normal eGFR is generally over 90, although many people may have an eGFR below this. A level below 60, however, is definitely indicative of some impairment of kidney function. The blood test should be performed at least once a year.

The other test of kidney function is a urine test to assess the amount of a protein called albumin in the urine. Albumin is a protein found in the blood and while the kidney should normally excrete creatinine into the urine, it should not excrete albumin. There is normally only a very small amount of albumin found in the urine. However, in diabetic kidney disease the blood capillaries become leaky, which means that substances such as albumin leak through into the urine. While this is not a good thing, it does provide a simple means of checking whether the kidneys are working properly. All that this test requires is that you collect a sample of urine that is sent to a laboratory to have the level of albumin and of creatinine measured. The result is expressed as the albumin to creatinine ratio (or ACR for short). A level of up to 3.5 is generally considered normal. If your test result is higher than this, it does not necessarily mean that you have diabetic kidney disease as there are a number of other factors that may cause a higher level (e.g. a urinary infection or increased physical activity).

My general recommendation is that if the result is above 3.5 then two further urine samples should be taken first thing in the morning. Very often these will be normal; however, if the levels are consistently raised then this suggests that the kidneys have been affected by diabetes.

A slightly raised level (e.g. up to 30) is termed microalbuminuria (literally, 'small amount of albumin in the urine'). If you are diagnosed with microalbuminuria, you will usually be prescribed medication to reduce the pressure in the kidneys. The usual treatment is an ACE inhibitor, such as Ramipril, which is also used to treat high blood pressure. This, together with better control of glucose and blood pressure, can help reduce the albumin leak, sometimes to normal levels.

Higher levels of ACR are termed macroalbuminuria. This will also require treatment with an ACE inhibitor. This may not improve the albumin leak, but will usually prevent further damage. Without treatment, however, diabetic kidney disease can progress to cause scarring of the kidneys, high blood pressure and eventually kidney failure. Fortunately, this is now rare in people with type 2 diabetes. However, there are no symptoms associated with albumin in the urine, and, as with the other checks mentioned in this chapter, it is vitally important to get the urine test done, so that if there is evidence of diabetes affecting your kidneys, appropriate treatment can be started in order to prevent more serious damage.

OTHER HEALTH CHECKS

The other checks required are a measure of blood pressure and a blood test to check cholesterol levels as in the previous chapter. These can be done at the same time as the eGFR blood test. Sometimes other tests will be added, such as a check on thyroid hormone levels (an underactive thyroid is a very common problem and makes it difficult to lose weight) or liver function tests. Liver tests are often abnormal as a result of fat in the liver that we now understand is part of the problem in causing insulin resistance in type 2 diabetes. If fatty liver affects you, then your liver blood tests should improve as you adopt the changes recommended in this book and lose weight.

It is quite common for these yearly checks to be done together in the form of annual review. Ideally, you should have all the results available so that you can discuss them with your diabetes team who will help you understand their significance, and so that you can participate in the decisions about, and fully comprehend the need for, any treatment or lifestyle changes. This is a process that is called care planning. National guidance suggests that this should be a collaborative process during which the person with diabetes plays a full and informed role.[2] My hope is that the knowledge you have gained by reading this book will enable you to do just that.

CHAPTER 18

STOP SMOKING

Everyone knows it. In fact even hardened smokers know it: smoking is seriously bad for your health. Although smoking is gradually declining in the UK, it still remains a major public health problem, contributing to thousands of deaths every year from heart disease and lung cancer. When we ran the Focus education programme in Bournemouth, we collected data on everyone when they were first diagnosed with type 2 diabetes. Ten years ago we found that around 15 per cent of people were smokers at the time they were diagnosed, a number we considered encouragingly low. However, recent national figures suggest that not much has changed since, with one in six people with diabetes (17 per cent) being smokers.

As discussed in chapter 3 smoking increases the risk of vascular (blood vessel) disease. As does diabetes. So the two really do not mix. It is therefore important that everyone with diabetes who smokes is offered support to help them stop smoking, as, over time, this will significantly reduce the risk of future health problems. If you do smoke, I am sure you are aware of the various methods available to help you stop smoking. These include support from stop smoking advisors, nicotine replacement therapy (available in various forms such as patches, lozenges, mouth spray) and medication designed to reduce cravings. All have been shown to help people give up smoking and are generally safe for people with diabetes.

A relatively new development has seen the marketing of so-called e-cigarettes, which look like cigarettes and release a small amount of nicotine vapour. These are not yet regulated as medical products and although there is evidence they can be effective at helping people stop smoking,[1] there is concern that their marketing may encourage continued smoking.

Whatever way you choose to go about stopping, it is important to appreciate that you are very unlikely to succeed in giving up smoking unless you really want to, and you are sufficiently motivated to persevere through the cravings and other withdrawal symptoms you will probably experience. It is also important to know that few people succeed in giving up smoking permanently on their first attempt. Most people who succeed have tried at least five times before they finally quit. So the moral is, if you do not succeed, try, try and try again. And when you do succeed, your health will benefit enormously. I recently found this fascinating article on a Canadian website that lists all the benefits from the day you stop until 15 years later:[2]

Here are some other good things that happen to your body once you stop smoking:

- Within 8 hours: carbon monoxide level drops in your body; oxygen level in your blood increases to normal.
- Within 48 hours: your chances of having a heart attack start to go down; your sense of smell and taste begin to improve.
- Within 72 hours: your bronchial tubes relax, making breathing easier; your lung capacity increases.
- Within two weeks to three months: your blood circulation improves; your lung functioning increases up to 30 per cent.
- Within six months: your coughing, stuffy nose, tiredness and shortness of breath all improve.
- Within one year: your risk of smoking-related heart attack is cut in half.
- Within 10 years: your risk of dying from lung cancer is cut in half.

- Within 15 years: your risk of dying from a heart attack is the same as a person who never smoked.

There are many other good reasons to quit smoking:

- You'll set a good example for your children.
- Your smoking will no longer affect the health of people around you.
- You'll have more money to save or to spend on other things – a pack of cigarettes a day adds up to £2,900 a year!
- You'll have more energy to do the things you love doing.
- You'll pay lower life insurance premiums.
- Cigarettes will no longer control your life.

So if you do smoke, understand this: you are not helping yourself and your health will definitely benefit from stopping smoking. I would plead with you to consider quitting.

However, as with all the lifestyle changes I have suggested to help you manage your diabetes, it is important that the process of stopping smoking is going to be a realistic and manageable change for you. That, in turn, will depend on a number of factors, including your motivation and what else is going on in your life. The danger is that if you try to stop smoking at the same time as you try to cut down on some of your favourite foods and increase your activity levels, you will not succeed at any of them – and will quickly become hugely disheartened. Therefore, while I strongly dislike everything to do with cigarette smoking, I always advise people with diabetes to concentrate on their diabetes management, or their weight management first, and once they have succeeded in making the changes to their diet and activity levels, then to consider stopping smoking. The reasons for this advice are:

1. Stopping smoking can be associated with weight gain, especially if you find it difficult to control what you eat. It is better to work on changing your diet first as this is key to losing weight and controlling your diabetes. Making progress with this will not only make you feel good in yourself, it will hopefully increase your motivation to stop smoking. By now you will have learned to control what you eat, so that when you do experience cravings for cigarettes you will be less likely to hit sugary foods in their place.

2. If your blood glucose levels are high you are likely to feel below par and at times unwell. This will not make it easy for you to stop smoking. If your glucose levels are very high, the immediate and greater risk to your health will come from uncontrolled diabetes.

Either way, you are more likely to be able to stick with changes that reduce your glucose levels (and make you feel better) than with stopping smoking, which initially may make you feel worse.

3. If you are newly diagnosed with type 2 diabetes it is very important that you learn to make appropriate changes to your diet as soon as possible, as the earlier and the better the initial improvements to your glucose levels, the better the longer-term outlook. Unless you are superhuman, this will require all your willpower and motivation, without the distraction of trying to stop smoking at the same time.

In chapter 21 we will discuss the importance of setting your own goals to help you reverse diabetes. If you do smoke I hope that stopping smoking will be one of your goals. However, the timing of that goal is up to you and it is entirely reasonable to concentrate on the immediate goals that will help you reverse diabetes the quickest.

CHAPTER 19

GETTING SUPPORT AND EDUCATION

In this book I have set out to describe how type 2 diabetes typically results from how modern-day living leads us to consume too much of the wrong types of food and drink, and to spending too much of our time inactive. The key to reversing diabetes is to reverse these behaviours, specifically to make changes to what we eat and drink, and to increase activity levels. Some people may only need to make small changes, which they may find they can accomplish quite quickly and easily. For others, even making small changes may prove difficult. And for some, where a greater degree of change is required, they may find the task nigh on impossible. This is why it is so important that, as you embark on making lifestyle changes, you are supported as much as possible by the people around you, whether it's your family or your diabetes team. And by having the right information to help you plan and make the most appropriate and effective changes.

It has long been recognised that the successful management of diabetes is largely down to patient self-management as pretty much everything someone does can affect his or her blood glucose levels. So it is important that anyone with diabetes receives an appropriate and targeted education designed to teach him or her how best to manage his or her diabetes. In 2000 the first ever National Service Framework for Diabetes in England was published by the Department of Health.[1] It stipulated that everyone with diabetes should receive self-management education at the time of diagnosis and at intervals thereafter. Since then there has been a big increase in education programmes for people with type 2 diabetes. Many areas run programmes developed locally for their own population. There are also so-called national programmes, which are run in many different areas across the country. The two national programmes for people with type 2 diabetes are X-Pert[2] and DESMOND[3] (which is an acronym for 'diabetes education and self management for ongoing and newly diagnosed').

X-Pert was developed by Dr Trudi Deakin while working as a dietitian in the north of England (dietitians are experts in food and nutrition who advise people on what to eat in order to lead a healthy lifestyle or achieve a specific health-related goal). It runs for six sessions at weekly intervals with a focus on the importance of diet in managing diabetes. When compared with the experiences of people who have not attended the programme, X-Pert has been shown to have a significant beneficial effect in helping people achieve better control of their diabetes without the need for so much medication. To my mind, better control with less medication means there has been some reversal of diabetes – even in those who have had the condition for several years.

DESMOND, on the other hand, is delivered as a single session on one day. It is designed to introduce people with newly diagnosed type 2 diabetes to the changes they can make to help control their diabetes. A trial conducted in 2008 to determine its effectiveness reached the conclusion that DESMOND resulted in greater improvements in weight loss and smoking cessation and positive improvements in beliefs about illness, but no difference in HbA1c levels compared to those who did not participate in DESMOND.[3]

Local programmes generally run over a few weeks. The Focus education programme, which has run in Bournemouth for over 20 years, comprises three sessions spread over a four- to six-week period. This gives people time between sessions to implement changes and to observe their effects. The majority of participants achieved very good control of their diabetes over the next few months, without any medication – demonstrating that it is the changes to lifestyle, predominantly diet, that has had this effect. It also highlights how the right information at the time of diagnosis can be very effective in helping people make the changes that will facilitate his or her control of the condition – and ultimately reverse it.

Going back in time, in the 1970s and 1980s, a large trial took place in many centres across the UK (the United Kingdom Prospective Diabetes Study or UKPDS), in which all subjects received dietary advice from a dietitian three times in the first few weeks after they were diagnosed with diabetes. During this period of the study no one was started on any medication. After three months there was a big improvement in their overall diabetic control, as measured by their HbA1c.

If one compares the effects of different types of education received after diagnosis, it appears that they all achieve a similar improvement in glucose control. This suggests that, soon after diagnosis, it is relatively easy to help people make changes that will improve his or her diabetic control. This may be because at this stage people are motivated to make changes; it may also be that small changes at the outset can have quite a marked effect, which appears to last for about three years according to an analysis carried out at Bournemouth.[4] So, while such programmes may be helpful in introducing people to the changes they can make to help control their diabetes, these changes need to continue into the long term, and that is where support is so often lacking. If, as often happens, glucose levels then start to rise, the traditional response has been (and still is) to prescribe medication, and as we saw in the last chapter, some of these may make it almost impossible to reverse diabetes.

It is also true that most education programmes are based on the traditional dietary advice that so many people find simply does not work, and are based on the 'eatwell plate'[5] that recommends a diet rich in starchy carbohydrates and includes fruit juice as both a healthy option and one of the five-a-day. Theoretically, and depending on how literally people take it, this advice may in itself lead to the subsequent deterioration in control of diabetes that many people experience. Furthermore, many education programmes still present diabetes as being a progressive incurable disease (as was thought to be the case until the last few years). Not only is this now known to be factually incorrect, it is also a message lacking in hope. To repeat what I have already said: there is a genuine chance of reversing diabetes if the right lifestyle changes are made at the outset. I do not think this new and transformational emphasis should be underestimated.

Personally, if I, as a newly diagnosed patient, were to be presented with diabetes as a progressive condition that I can, at best, control, but which will never go away, my motivation to make (possibly challenging) lifestyle changes would be far lower than if I were presented with the evidence that, if I make the right changes, I might potentially free myself from diabetes and its associated health risks.

Another issue in the UK is that despite the big increase in the provision of education programmes, there are still many geographical areas where no programmes are available, or where there are too few places for the number of people who are developing diabetes. Given the rapid increase in obesity and in type 2 diabetes, it is questionable whether health services will ever be able to keep up with the demand by providing enough face-to-face education.

That is one of the reasons why I decided to write this book – to ensure above all that someone who is newly diagnosed with type 2 diabetes has accurate and up-to-date information about the lifestyle changes that will help reverse diabetes. If you have read this far the chances are you already have a pretty good idea of what you can do to help reverse your diabetes, and you may not gain much more from attending an education programme. However, for people who find it less easy to learn by reading a book, I would definitely recommend attending an education programme, although its recommendations may differ in some ways from mine.

Most programmes are one-offs, lasting from one to six sessions. While they may be effective in providing access to the right information early on, this is just the start. Success depends on being able to make changes and to stick to them. Given that type 2 diabetes requires lifestyle change first and foremost, it would be logical for the health service to provide ongoing support and education to help people maintain these changes, yet that is rarely the case. There are excellent examples elsewhere in Europe, notably in Italy, where ongoing education is provided to small groups of people.[6] Given that everyone with type 2 diabetes is reviewed at their GP's surgery on a regular basis, it should be feasible to use the same time and resources to provide a more educationally based service, rather than seeing everyone individually. However, I am aware of only very few practices which have actually tried to do this.

The other benefit from attending a programme is that you will have the chance to meet other people in the same position as yourself, something many people find extremely helpful. Not only is it reassuring to know that there are others in a very similar situation to you, you will often learn from other people's experiences, and get a chance to try something out when you have seen that it has worked for someone else.

The Internet is a great place for people with diabetes to access support. There are several UK-based sites that offer good-quality information for people with diabetes, and also forums for people to exchange information and ideas. Although there is no guarantee that the advice given will work for any one individual, or indeed that it is accurate, I have been extremely impressed with the quality of advice provided through some of these forums. I have no hesitation in recommending them to anyone who wishes to draw on the experience of other people with diabetes, particularly when it comes trying out different ideas regarding food and exercise. Of course you should never make any changes to your medication without discussing it with your doctor or diabetes nurse first. Such forums also provide an opportunity for people to share experiences and concerns about their diabetes. There will always be someone else who has had the same sort of experience and who may have found a way through it and is willing to share it with you.

See appendix 1 for a list of useful websites.

Making lifestyle changes is always easier with someone else's help and support, rather than trying to do it all on your own. It can be very difficult attempting to change your diet while others in your house continue to eat the very foods you are trying to avoid. That isn't to say that everyone else should go without cakes and biscuits (though in many cases it would be good for them too!), but if they are willing to make some changes along with you it will certainly help. Or maybe you have a friend who is also keen to make changes to their lifestyle with whom you could go walking or join an exercise class or sports club together, and in this way provide support for each other. Joining a slimming club or an exercise class will not only help you towards your goal, but the discipline of having to turn up every week can be a very motivating factor, especially if you will be weighed. Hopefully you will also make new friends through such a group – another benefit from the activity.

If you do your own cooking and shopping then you are already in control of what you eat, and you can start the process of change by buying and cooking different foods. If you rely on someone else to do this for you, it is essential that they are on board with, and fully understand, the changes you want and need to make. It is worth taking the time to explain in some detail how you plan to change your diet so that they understand why you no longer wish to eat big portions of pasta or mashed potato. Just as the changes may be difficult for you, the change can be equally difficult for the person who has to start preparing different types of meals. You may like to show them the boxed section of this chapter (below) as a means of explaining this to them.

INFORMATION FOR FRIENDS OR RELATIVES

If you live with, or care for, someone with diabetes, then you will be aware of the many demands that the condition places on that person, and probably on you as well. The aim of this book is to help people with type 2 diabetes take control of their condition more effectively in order to reverse the disease processes that cause diabetes. Now that statement may come as a surprise to you, as it was previously believed that once you had type 2 diabetes you had it for life.

This has now been shown to be untrue.

Rather, it appears that diabetes results from excess fat accumulating in the liver and the pancreas, and that by making changes to the diet this fat can be reduced, thus reversing the disease. In many cases this enables the person with diabetes to control the condition with less medication, and in some cases, the diabetes disappears altogether.

The main problem in type 2 diabetes is that the body cannot use insulin properly. This leads to the pancreas producing extra insulin, resulting in the levels of insulin in the blood rising too high. As insulin is the main 'fat hormone' this leads to more fat being laid down in the internal organs, which makes the problem even worse.

It is known that losing weight and getting more active can help reduce insulin levels. Therefore, the key changes that need to be made are to the diet and to activity levels. Specifically, it is important to reduce the amount of carbohydrate (sugar and starch) in the diet. This is because all carbohydrates cause the level of glucose (sugar) in the blood to rise, and also cause the release of insulin into the bloodstream. Reducing carbohydrates therefore helps directly by keeping the blood glucose level stable, and avoids high insulin levels. Over time, as insulin levels reduce, it will result in the loss of fat from the liver. Insulin can again work more efficiently in controlling sugar levels, which in turn means the body does not release so much of it into the bloodstream, and so on, leading to a virtuous circle of positive health benefits.

So what does this mean on a day-to-day basis? Put simply, it means reducing the amount of bread, potatoes, rice, pasta, cereals and sweet foods and drinks (including fruit juice and some fruit) in the diet. So the person with diabetes is going to be helped by having only very small portions of these foods, and will benefit from having some meals with none of these foods in them at all. I realise this may be very different from what you were told in the past – that people with diabetes should eat starchy carbohydrates with every meal. Quite simply that approach has not worked, whereas more and more people, including many that I have treated, have found that restricting carbohydrates really does work.

Note that I am saying, 'restrict carbohydrates'. I certainly do not suggest stopping them altogether. However, a breakfast based on eggs or plain yoghurt is better than cereals. A salad or soup with or without a small piece of bread is better than sandwiches or a baguette for lunch. And for other meals, keeping the starchy food (potato, pasta or rice) to a small portion of the plate and using lots of leafy vegetables will certainly help.

The other change that will help is increasing physical activity. This does not necessarily mean going to the gym regularly, but can consist of trying to use the car less, and walking or using public transport more. It can mean going for a walk every day, and, importantly, avoiding sitting down continuously for long periods of time (e.g. in front of the television or at a computer). Even getting up and walking around for a few minutes every hour or so will help.

I have noticed that people seem to do very well when their partner or a close friend supports them, especially when they join in making some of the same changes. In many cases their own health improves as well and that can't be a bad thing! I am sure that the person who asked you to read this will be very grateful for your help in supporting them in making these changes. If you are interested, you will find more detailed information in chapters 6 to 12.

Successful management of diabetes means effective self-management, as the person with diabetes can influence their diabetes by the choices they make in respect of what they eat and how active they are. Making appropriate choices requires that the person with diabetes has the right information and skills to make appropriate changes, and the support necessary to maintain them.

That is the fundamental aim of this book: to ensure that you have accurate and up-to-date information about the lifestyle changes, which will help control and reverse your diabetes.

I hope that the later chapters in this book will help you decide what changes you can make, and provide you with some advice about how to make those changes part of your new life. Keeping the book handy for future reference will mean you can remind yourself of key pieces of information at any time in the future.

CHAPTER 20

REVERSING DIABETES DISTRESS

From the preceding chapters you will have learnt how having type 2 diabetes can affect many aspects of daily living – both as a result of the disease itself or because of health problems related to your diabetes or because you must undertake a series of lifestyle changes needed to manage your diabetes. You will also have learnt how everyday activities can affect type 2 diabetes, especially concerning food intake and activity levels. And we have discussed how illness can also affect diabetes. In short: type 2 diabetes can affect many aspects of everyday life, and many aspects of everyday life can affect type 2 diabetes. It is little wonder, therefore, that at times having type 2 diabetes can cause stress, anxiety and even depression. In addition, a person with diabetes may have psychological issues that are unrelated to their diabetes. Regardless of its cause, stress, anxiety or depression can all impact on a person's ability to manage their diabetes.

For a long time, it has been recognised that people with diabetes are more likely to experience anxiety and depression than people without diabetes. More recently it has been recognised that having diabetes is a major cause of psychological ill health, and the term 'diabetes distress' has been introduced to describe the emotional and psychological effects experienced by people with diabetes. As diabetes distress is associated with higher HbA1c levels,[1] and increased risk of diabetes-related complications, there is growing recognition that it needs to be taken more seriously.

The DAWN2 study[2] was a large study that was undertaken in 17 countries around the world in 2011. It looked specifically at the psychological, educational and emotional needs of people with diabetes and came up with some very interesting results. Nearly half of all people with diabetes reported high levels of diabetes distress and one in seven people had such low emotional well-being that they were likely to be suffering from depression. The study also found that diabetes had a negative impact on family and other relationships, on leisure activities, work and finances. So what causes diabetes distress?

Diabetes distress is likely to result from a number of factors that affect people with the disease. These include how well they accept the diagnosis of diabetes, how they adjust to the lifestyle changes required to control it, and how they cope with complications if they arise. Even in the absence of long-term complications, just having high blood glucose levels can affect mood or the ability to concentrate, as well as cause unpleasant physical symptoms such as thirst, frequent urination and erectile dysfunction. These readily explain how having diabetes can affect relationships, family life and employment. It is also easy to imagine how someone, burdened by these problems, might find it more difficult to make the changes to their diet and lifestyle that are needed to control their diabetes. Indeed, diabetes distress has been shown to be associated with lower levels of physical activity, poor diet and reduced adherence to prescribed treatments. This in turn explains why diabetes distress is associated with worse control of diabetes, which in turn increases the risk of complications, which in themselves will likely further exacerbate diabetes distress – creating a vicious circle as shown below.

THE DIABETES DISTRESS VICIOUS CIRCLE

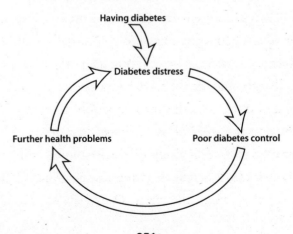

A number of studies have shown that the way people are managed when they are first diagnosed with diabetes creates a significant mental impression and it's something that stays with them for many years.[3] Not only does it impact on a person's diabetes control and physical health, but also on his or her psychological health. For many people being diagnosed with diabetes comes as a nasty shock – and may be associated with a number of different emotions.

- **Fear:** if they know someone who has suffered from diabetes in the past, especially if that individual had a bad time with it
- **Resentment:** if they resent their loss of health and the consequent freedom to eat and do whatever they want
- **Isolation:** if they happen to be the only one among family and friends to have diabetes
- **Guilt:** if they think that diabetes results from their own actions, such as gaining too much weight
- **Confusion:** if they have been given inappropriate advice on what they should or should not eat, perhaps from a well-meaning relative
- **Helplessness:** if they believe their diabetes will gradually get worse, regardless of what they do

Some of these powerful emotions are the product of the thoughts, feelings and worries that naturally emerge within the person who is newly diagnosed, but others arise from the things that are communicated by people around them, who may previously have had second-hand experiences of other people's diabetes. Regardless of their origin, I believe it is important that everyone at diagnosis of diabetes has an opportunity to express their feelings, and to receive high-quality education about how they can best manage their diabetes going forward. Getting the right information at the beginning can help correct any misinformation that may lead to negative emotions. Until recently, even giving accurate information may still have caused negative emotions, as it was believed that type 2 diabetes was always permanent and over time would gradually and inevitably and get worse. Put crudely, the message was, 'you have it for life, it will get gradually worse, but you can make changes that can slow down how quickly it gets worse'. For some people, who for whatever reason may be poorly motivated or rather despondent in their outlook on life, this could lead to a feeling of 'whatever I do won't make that much difference, so I might as well get on and enjoy myself'. But we now know that type 2 diabetes can be reversed – and that should make all the difference as we set the tone and nature of the initial educational framework.

To be clear, we are still a long way from knowing precisely to what extent type 2 diabetes can be reversed and in how many people, but the unarguable truth is that the physical and metabolic changes associated with diabetes are not permanent and can be reversed. To my mind this is essential information for anyone newly diagnosed with type 2 diabetes. Knowing that diabetes can be reversed could fundamentally affect how many people respond in terms of the effort they put in to make the necessary changes to their lifestyle. It also provides a message of hope and of empowerment: changes you make can and will help you improve your health. If conveyed correctly, I believe that this could lead to a lot less diabetes distress arising at the time of diagnosis.

Another source of diabetes distress arises from the traditional advice about how diabetes should be managed with its emphasis on medication rather than lifestyle, coupled with its guidance on diet that may actually be counter-productive. Both risk increasing feelings of helplessness in the person with diabetes. The reliance on medication risks neglecting the potential for the person to take control of their condition, especially if that medication leads to weight gain. A carbohydrate-rich diet, despite containing 'healthy' carbohydrates, risks causing high blood glucose levels, and further risks causing confusion and despondency in someone who believes they are doing 'the right thing'. I would therefore anticipate that a more emphatic focus on lifestyle changes as the main means of controlling diabetes, coupled with a simple explanation about which foods will help keep blood glucose levels under control, will help people feel they are in control of their condition. This will in turn reduce feelings of helplessness and of anxiety.

The DAWN2 study showed that people who received education about their diabetes felt better equipped to manage their diabetes, were more actively involved in their care, received more support and reported better well-being. It is recognised that access to good-quality information about diabetes, as well as self-management education, can help reduce anxiety related to diabetes. Modern education programmes place an emphasis not just on how to manage diabetes, but also in developing goal-setting, problem-solving and coping skills, so that when things go wrong, as occasionally they will, the individual is well equipped to deal with them. This highlights the importance of self-management education in helping reduce diabetes distress.

The long-term complications of diabetes are an obvious source of diabetes distress. Experiencing loss of vision, a foot ulcer or erectile dysfunction will inevitably be a cause of huge anxiety. When complications arise it is right that the immediate priority is given to the medical treatments that will help manage the complication. However, it is important that the person with diabetes, as well as his or her health-care team, recognise the emotional effects complications may have on their mental well-being. He or she should also be provided with both support and appropriate treatment for any mental distress. If you are in this situation, and you feel you have not been offered appropriate support, please discuss it with someone in your diabetes team.

Specialists in the field of diabetes psychology rank the various types of psychological problem from the mildest, which are very common (level 1), to the most severe, which are, fortunately, very rare (level 5).[4] Level 1 includes general difficulties with coping with diabetes and its effects on lifestyle. These are the sorts of problems that can be greatly helped by self-management education, either individually or as part of a group. Receiving training in coping strategies, and securing peer support from other people with diabetes, can also help. Level 2 includes more severe difficulties in coping with diabetes that can cause significant anxiety or low mood, and can affect the individual's ability to manage their diabetes. These types of problems require more specific treatment, such as cognitive behavioural therapy (CBT) or a course of treatment with an antidepressant, such as paroxetine.

Level 3 problems include binge-eating disorder, which is common in people with type 2 diabetes. This is an eating disorder characterised by out of control over-eating (binge-eating) that often leads to weight gain. It is likely that diabetes results from the weight gain, although other factors may also be involved. It requires specialised psychological treatment such as CBT.

At the end of the scale (level 5) are certain types of severe mental illness that are associated with diabetes. These include bipolar disorder (manic-depression) and schizophrenia. Sufferers of both of these conditions have a greater risk of diabetes than normal. It is not known for certain why this is the case: diabetes may result from the difficulties these illnesses can cause that prevent a sufferer from maintaining a healthy lifestyle, or from biochemical changes which predispose an individual to both diabetes and these mental conditions themselves, or from the effect of drugs used to treat them – or a combination of all of these. These conditions are rare and require specialist treatment that falls outside the scope of this book.

As the aim of this book is to provide you with the tools to manage your diabetes, my hope is that any diabetes distress you may have experienced will reduce with time once you learn how you can take control of, and begin to reverse, your diabetes. In other words the diabetes distress should reverse with the reversal of diabetes. However, if you continue to experience anxiety or low-mood relating to your diabetes, or to another problem, please seek help.

Depression makes it more difficult to make changes to diet or activity levels. Therefore, it is likely that if you are depressed you will find it far more challenging to make the changes necessary to control your diabetes; the depression may need to be treated first.

The National Institute for Health and Care Excellence (NICE) states that health-care professionals working in diabetes teams should be alert to the development or presence of depression or anxiety, especially in people who find it difficult to manage their diabetes. They should also be able to detect and manage non-severe psychological disorders, and have access to more specialist psychological services for the more complex problems. Unfortunately, in a recent survey conducted by Diabetes UK, only 32 per cent of diabetes services had access to specialist psychological provision.[5] However, this must not put you off seeking treatment if you need it.

In summary, diabetes distress is a very common problem, arising from different aspects of having diabetes.

It can result in negative emotions, anxiety and low mood, which make it difficult to manage diabetes. Ensuring you are properly educated in how to manage your diabetes and knowing how to deal with setbacks when they arise can all help improve diabetes distress although more severe symptoms may require psychological or medical treatments. The aim of this book is to provide the education you need to manage your diabetes, and it is my hope that reading this book, knowing that diabetes can be reversed, and seeing the benefits of lifestyle changes you make, will all help reduce any diabetes distress you may experience.

CHAPTER 21

SETTING YOUR OWN GOALS, MAKING CHANGES AND STICKING TO THEM

If you have read this book from the beginning you will now understand and, I hope, believe the simple fact that type 2 diabetes can be reversed. You may already have a clear idea of the steps you can take in order to help control and reverse your diabetes. These can be broadly classified as:

1. Changes to your diet
2. Changes to your lifestyle
3. Changes to your treatment

Life is full of good intentions, many of which, if we're honest with ourselves, are never realised. Therefore, it is important that if you are about to make significant lifestyle changes, you set yourself realistic goals. It is equally important to be honest with yourself about how motivated you are to make these changes. Reading this book probably hasn't been your idea of fun. I sincerely hope, though, that most of it will have been interesting. But the fact that you have read the book through to this point suggests that you are at least sufficiently motivated to find out what you can do to improve your health, and I take that as a positive sign: you are going to be motivated to make some important changes in your life.

If, for whatever reason, you have jumped straight to this chapter, I would strongly suggest you start at the beginning of the book and work your way through it. It will give you an idea about what changes you can realistically make. And if that seems too much like hard work, maybe you should put the book on a shelf (preferably somewhere where you can find it again!) until you do feel motivated to have a crack at reading it.

If you have read through from the beginning, there is a good chance that you have already made some changes. If you have not yet done so, maybe you are actively considering making some changes in the next few weeks. If so, read on. If you still do not feel ready to make changes in the next few weeks, it is unlikely that you will be able to keep them up, and I would suggest waiting until you do feel ready before committing to change.

Here, I want to point out that there is absolutely nothing wrong with not being ready to make changes. It is human nature that we all do the things we think are important for us right now. If, at the moment, you do not think it is important to make a change, then it's probably not worth trying, you will be setting yourself up to fail. That isn't the same thing as saying you do not understand how a change may be beneficial to your health, rather it is an acknowledgement that your current lifestyle, which perhaps includes a family or work situation that is consuming all of your energy, is more important to you right now.

We have already debated the merits of giving up cigarette smoking. Isn't it extraordinary how everyone knows how truly awful the habit is for his or her immediate and long-term well-being, and yet people continue to smoke (17 per cent of those newly diagnosed with diabetes smoke, as I have stated earlier). The enjoyment people get from smoking (coupled with its addictive nature) proves to be more attractive than the processes of trying to give up something pleasurable now in order to derive health benefits in the future. The key is always – how ready are you to change? In order for you to assess this, it might be helpful to ask yourself two questions:

1. On a scale of zero (not at all important) to ten (extremely important), how important is it for me to make changes to help reverse my diabetes?
2. On a scale of zero (not at all confident) to ten (extremely confident), how confident do I feel that I can make changes to help reverse my diabetes?

In my clinical experience, most people to whom I put these questions give a high score (usually eight, nine or ten) to the first question. After all, they have chosen to come to see me to discuss their diabetes. However, the answers to the second question would usually vary quite a lot. If your answer to both questions is high (and you are being honest in your assessment!), then you are ready to change. However, if your answer to the second question is four or five, then you should follow it up with some further questions:

3. What is the reason or reasons I chose to score so low to the second question?
4. What would need to happen for me to be able to give myself a higher score?

This may prompt you to focus on what are the barriers to you making the changes to lifestyle including diet and levels of physical activity and addressing those barriers so that you are better able to make the changes.

If you are still with me I am assuming you feel that now is the time to have a go and to make some changes in your lifestyle. And so before going any further, I would like to return to the questions that were posed at the end of chapter 7. Even if you have answered them earlier, please spend some time now answering them as fully as you can. Write your answers down; it will be useful to refer to them in the future:

- What are your reasons for reading this book?
- What frustrates you most about having diabetes?
- How do you want things to be different?
- How will you know when you have achieved this?
- What is the main thing you would like to change after reading this book?

Your answer to the last question is the main goal you have just set yourself.

It doesn't really matter what the goal is, as long as you are ready to make some changes to achieve it. It may be a relatively small goal, such as stopping drinking fruit juice. In this case the change you need to make is quite obvious, and I would recommend that you ask yourself the questions on the previous page about how ready you are to make this change, to check it is achievable, and then to go for it. If you are successful this will spur you on to set yourself further challenges and goals.

It may be, however, that you set yourself quite a significant goal, such as no longer having diabetes. In this case I would recommend that you break it down into specific changes that you feel you can make in order to ultimately achieve your goal – and to write them down. Alongside each one write the scores to the two 'readiness to change' questions, and then add them up and put them in the final column. You will end up with something like this:

My goal is: _____

In order to do this I will aim to:

The Change	How important is it for me to do it? (0–10 scale)	How confident am I that I can do it? (0–10 scale)	Sum of both scores

I would suggest that right now, before going any further, you take some time to list the most realistic changes you can make to help you achieve your goal. If you need to read through some of the earlier chapters then do so, but please do it as soon as you can – and only read on once you have done it.

You will now have a table that looks something like this:

My goal is: to reduce my blood glucose levels

In order to do this I will aim to:

Change	How important is it for me to do it? (0–10 scale)	How confident am I that I can do it? (0–10 scale)	Sum of both scores
Stop drinking fruit juice	10	10	20
Walk round the block five times a week	10	7	17
Go to the gym	7	3	10
Walk to work	7	6	13
Stop eating breakfast cereals	8	6	14
Eat less bread	9	8	17
Eat more vegetables	9	8	17

In theory the change with the highest score is the one that you will find easiest to do followed by the one with the next highest score. So in this example the first thing to do will be to throw away (or give away if unopened) all the fruit juice you have in the house. Now this may be less easy if you live with someone who craves fruit juice every day, in which case you may need to manage your change in a less drastic way, but the point is you need to do something to show you and those around you how determined you are. Then make sure you have enough vegetables in the house to fulfil your next planned change of eating more vegetables. And decide what time of day you will go for a walk round the block – when it is most likely you will actually manage to do it. It may be helpful to write down your top three changes, and how you will achieve them:

Change	How will I achieve this?	When will I start
Stop drinking fruit juice	Stop buying it; tell everyone I no longer drink it	Today
Walk round the block five times a week	Go after evening meal	Next week
Eat more vegetables	Buy frozen green beans, and fresh carrots	Today

Once you have achieved these changes then you can consider addressing the next item on your list and so on. You don't necessarily have to go through this process with every change you plan to make, but it may be helpful to start with. The aim is that you only plan to make changes that are SMART. That is:

Specific: so you know exactly what you are going to do
Measurable: you know how to tell if you have achieved it
Achievable: it has to be a change that you are able to make
Realistic: one which you have a realistic chance of making
Timely: and one for which you can specify a time of making it

Please note that the changes I have used in this example are just examples. You have to be honest in choosing the ones that are the SMARTest ones for you.

Having chosen your schedule of changes, allow yourself occasional treats and relax the rules on special occasions. Why? Because if you really like fruit juice it may be difficult to contemplate a life where you never ever drink it again! But maybe you can live with having it as a treat once a week, especially if others in your household drink it and it is permanently in the fridge. But recognise that it will probably lead to your blood glucose level increasing – perhaps follow it up with a walk to help bring your blood glucose level down again.

Remember: you have developed your current eating and activity patterns over many years. Many of them will have become habits, behaviours that you follow because you always have done them. Some will be automatic, they are your 'default' way of behaving. It will not be easy to suddenly make a big change. As a general rule, therefore, you are more likely to achieve change in small steps. Don't try to commit to too many changes all at once. Small changes to your diet (or activity levels that you feel you are able to maintain) are more likely to help you achieve your goal than a drastic change that you cannot stick to for more than a couple of weeks. Success with your first small changes will give you the confidence to embark on some of the more difficult changes on your list.

Eating is a social activity, and if you make changes to the what, when or how you eat, it will impact on others

– especially those that you live with. So it helps to have others on board as you try to make changes. Maybe someone else in your household, or a close friend, could also do with making some changes to their diet or activity levels. Even if they do not have diabetes, the changes suggested here will help protect them from diabetes in the future. If there is no one else who is willing or able to make changes with you, it will help if there is someone who you can confide in, and who can support you as you start your programme of making changes and encourage you to stick with them.

At the end of the day, the success you have will depend on your own motivation to make changes, and your ability to stick to them. Over time motivation may well diminish, and everyday life will get in the way. What may be the high priority today (making changes to reverse your diabetes) may be superseded by a friend or family member becoming unwell, or a financial problem or just about anything else that life can throw at us. It is completely natural that daily living and the many crises that occur take your focus away from lifestyle changes. Be aware that as a result, you may slip back into your previous eating habits, or lower activity levels. If this does happen, please do not fall into the trap of blaming yourself or criticising yourself for failing.

Instead, focus on what you have achieved so far, and give yourself time to concentrate on the new priorities that have emerged in your life – without feelings of guilt.

However, if possible, see what changes you are able to maintain during this period, and whether it is possible to set yourself a plan to restart the other changes in the near future. If not, perhaps you can commit to reviewing your progress in four weeks' time, for example, even if you then decide you cannot make any further progress right now. It may be that rereading the goals you set yourself will help remotivate you. As might speaking to a trusted friend, or someone on your diabetes team.

Having completed the goal-setting exercise above, it may be helpful to recap some of the key components to taking control of – and reversing – your diabetes, to ensure your goals cover all the main points and that your lifestyle changes are as effective as possible in controlling your glucose levels.

1. You need to make changes to your diet. My recommendation is to adopt simple dietary changes as outlined in this book that mainly focus on reducing sugars and starches (including sugar-sweetened drinks). I know of many people who have used this approach to achieve significant weight loss and at least partial reversal of their diabetes. More drastic approaches, as used in Professor Taylor's research (see chapter 5) can also be used, and his team provides very helpful advice on how to adopt such a diet at the following address: http://www.ncl.ac.uk/magres/research/diabetes/documents/StudyRecipes.pdf. If you adopt

this approach, it is essential that you decide for how long you will take the diet, and decide what are the long-term changes you will make to ensure you do not put the weight back on. Remember that if you aim to lose a lot of weight it will be made easier if you avoid alcohol altogether for a while.

2. Would it help to discuss the changes you wish to make with a family member or a close friend? If you haven't already done so, show them the section for friends and relatives in chapter 19.

3. Alongside changes to the amount of calories you take in, you need to set some goals about using up more energy by increasing your activity levels. Remember that walking, cycling or using public transport is better than driving everywhere. Remember that getting up and walking around every hour is better than spending long periods of time in front of the television or computer. And that walking is one of the best exercises you can do. Is there any sport or other activity you would consider taking up?

4. If you take insulin or a sulfonylurea it is likely you will need to reduce the dose as you adopt these lifestyle changes. Please discuss the best approach with your diabetes team so that you minimise the risk of hypoglycaemia as a result of your current dose being too high for your new lifestyle.

5. Blood glucose monitoring is important in showing you how effective your lifestyle changes are in controlling your glucose levels. Remember that ideally they should be between 4 and 6mmol/l before meals, and no higher than 8mmol/l after meals. Make sure you have an up-to-date meter (most pharmacies sell a selection) and that you use it according to the manufacturer's instructions. Consider which of the types of monitoring discussed in chapter 13 would work best for you. How many strips will you need each month? Ask your GP if they will prescribe them for you. If not, consider buying them from a pharmacy or via diabetes.co.uk.

6. Be realistic about what you can achieve. It is quite likely that your body took years to undergo the changes that ultimately led to diabetes, so don't expect a miracle to happen overnight. It is far better to make steady changes that lead to gradual improvement over the course of weeks or months than to make drastic changes that you cannot sustain for more than a few days.

Finally, I would like to thank you for taking the trouble to read this book. The aim of the book has been to help you identify what changes you can make to help reverse your diabetes. The whole concept of reversing diabetes is relatively new, and we still do not know what proportion of people will be able to reverse their diabetes fully, or for how long. However, rather than waiting for the results of clinical trials to answer that question, I would encourage you to use the knowledge that type 2 diabetes can be reversed, to consider what changes you can make now to help promote the reversal of your own diabetes. Good luck!

ACKNOWLEDGEMENTS

First and foremost I wish to acknowledge the contribution of the thousands of people with type 2 diabetes, who over the years have taught me about the complexities and challenges that are part of living with type 2 diabetes. Thanks also to those from whom I learnt so much from their contributions to Internet discussion forums, especially on diabetes.co.uk and diabetes-support.org.uk, whose moderators have been so helpful in allowing me to ask questions of its members about their experiences living with diabetes. Thanks, too, to my own patients who in recent years were brave enough to try a different approach to their diet, which in many ways was very different from what they had previously been advised.

I am also hugely indebted to the amazing team at the Bournemouth Diabetes and Endocrine Centre, with whom I had the privilege of working for so many years, and who were always willing to try out new ideas in the quest to help people better manage their diabetes. I am particularly grateful to Emma Jenkins and Clare Shaban, who helped with specific sections of the book. Thanks also to Chris Cheyette who prepared the table on carbohydrate portion sizes, adapted from his *Carbs and Cals* book. I wish to acknowledge the pivotal role that

John Briffa had through his book *Escape the Diet Trap* in giving me the confidence to change my clinical practice, as well as some of my own dietary habits. Thank you to diabetes.co.uk, who suggested that I write the book, to Jonathan Hayden for encouraging me to do so and for making it happen. Thanks to my daughters Emma and Bex, and above all to my wife Mary, both for putting up with yet another of my 'projects' and also for encouraging me and showing interest in its progress along the way.

APPENDIX 1

USEFUL WEBSITES

Diabetes.co.uk

Diabetes.co.uk is the UK's largest and fastest-growing community website and forum for people with diabetes:
Get support at **www.diabetes.co.uk/forum**
Like us on Facebook **www.facebook.com/Diabetes.co.uk**
Sign up for FREE Newsletter **www.diabetes.co.uk/welcome**
Buy diabetes products and accessories online **www.diabetes.co.uk/shop**

Diabetes Support Forum UK

The diabetes-support.org.uk forum is open to ALL people who want to discuss diabetes, and everyone is very welcome, but our focus is mainly on the UK NHS system.
www.diabetes-support.org.uk

International Diabetes Federation

The global advocate for people with diabetes. The mission of IDF is to promote diabetes care, prevention and a cure worldwide.
www.idf.org

Diabetes UK

The UK's leading diabetes charity. They care for, connect with and campaign on behalf of all people affected by and at risk of diabetes in local communities across the UK.
www.diabetes.org.uk

NHS Choices

Information from the National Health Service on conditions, treatments, local services and healthy living.
www.nhs.uk/Conditions/Diabetes/Pages/Diabetes.aspx

Public Library of Science

Non-profit organization of scientists committed to making the world's scientific and medical literature freely accessible to scientists and to the public.
www.plos.org

Diabetes Community

An international community for people with diabetes.
www.diabetescommunity.com

Glycaemic index

www.glycemicindex.com

Carbs and Cals

Make carb and calorie counting easy to understand and accessible to everyone.
www.carbsandcals.com

Carbohydrate counting programme

Developed by the Bournemouth Diabetes and Endocrine Centre – mainly for people on insulin.
www.bdec-e-learning.com

The NHS Diabetic Eye Screening Programme (NDESP)

The NHS Diabetic Eye Screening Programme (NDESP) aims to reduce the risk of sight loss among people with diabetes by the early detection and treatment, if needed, of sight-threatening retinopathy.
diabeticeye.screening.nhs.uk

Patient Education programmes

www.nhs.uk/Livewell/Diabetes/Pages/Diabeteseducation.aspx

APPENDIX 2

BODY MASS INDEX GUIDANCE CHART

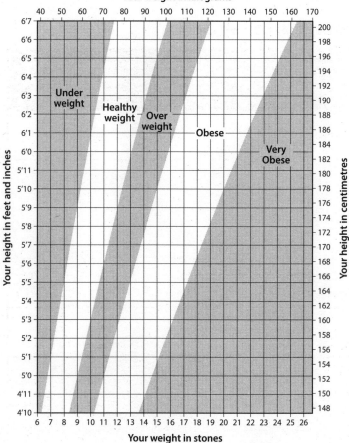

Your weight in kilograms

Your height in feet and inches

Your height in centimetres

- Under weight
- Healthy weight
- Over weight
- Obese
- Very Obese

Your weight in stones

APPENDIX 3

SIGNIFICANT GOALS AND READINESS TO CHANGE CHART

My goal is: _____

In order to do this I will aim to:

The Change	How important is it for me to do it? (0–10 scale)	How confident am I that I can do it? (0–10 scale)	Sum of both scores

GLOSSARY

ACE inhibitors: ACE inhibitors are a medication mainly used to lower blood pressure and the resulting strain on the heart and kidneys. ACE stands for angiotensin converting enzyme. Angiotensin is a chemical that can make blood vessels narrower to raise blood pressure.

Albuminuria: Damaged kidneys may start to leak protein into the urine. Albumin is a small, abundant protein in the blood that passes through the kidney filter into the urine more easily than other proteins. In people newly diagnosed with type 2 diabetes the kidneys may already show signs of small amounts of protein leakage called microalbuminuria. This may be because of diabetes or from other diseases seen in conjunction with diabetes such as high blood pressure. Protein in the urine increases the risk of developing kidney disease. It also means that the person is at a particularly high risk of the development of cardiovascular disease.

Alpha cells: Alpha cells are found in the islets of Langerhans in the pancreas. They produce and release glucagon.

Angiotensin II receptor antagonists: A class of drugs that work in a similar way to ACE inhibitors to reduce blood pressure. Angiotensin II receptor antagonists, also called angiotensin receptor blockers (ARBs), work by blocking the formation of angiotensin II, a substance that makes blood vessels narrower.

Antibodies: Proteins produced in the body that protect it from foreign substances such as bacteria or viruses.

Beta cells: Beta cells are found in the islets of Langerhans in the pancreas. They produce and release insulin.

Blood pressure: Blood pressure is the amount of force that is exerted by blood on the blood vessels. It is measured in millimetres of mercury (written as mm Hg). When blood pressure is taken the measurement is given as two numbers, for example 120/80mm Hg. The first number is called the systolic pressure and is the measure of pressure in the arteries when the heart beats and pushes more blood into the arteries. The second number, called the diastolic pressure, is the pressure in the arteries when the heart rests between beats. The ideal blood pressure for people with diabetes is less than 140/80.

Carbohydrate: A carbohydrate is a large organic molecule consisting of carbon (C), hydrogen (H) and oxygen (O) atoms. The term is most common in biochemistry, where it is synonymous with saccharide (sugar). The lighter versions of the molecules (monosaccharides and disaccharides) are commonly referred to as sugars. Carbohydrates perform numerous roles in living organisms including the storage of energy (e.g. starch and glycogen) and in an informal context, the term carbohydrate often means any food that is particularly rich in the complex carbohydrate starch (such as cereals, bread and pasta) or simple carbohydrates such as table sugar.

Cardiovascular disease (CVD): Cardiovascular diseases are defined as diseases and injuries of the circulatory system: the heart, the blood vessels of the heart and the system of blood vessels throughout the body and to (and in) the brain. Stroke is the result of a blood flow problem within, or leading to, the brain and is considered a form of CVD.

Cholesterol: A waxy substance made by the liver that is an essential part of cell walls and nerves. Cholesterol plays an important role in body functions such as digestion and hormone production. In addition to being produced by the body cholesterol comes from animal foods that we eat. Too much cholesterol in the blood causes an increase in particles called LDL ('bad' cholesterol), which increases the build-up of plaque in the artery walls and leads to atherosclerosis.

Diabetes complications: Diabetes complications are chronic conditions caused by diabetes. They include retinopathy (eye disease), nephropathy (kidney disease), neuropathy (nerve disease), cardiovascular disease (disease of the circulatory system), foot ulceration and amputation.

Diabetes mellitus (DM): Diabetes mellitus is a chronic condition that arises when the pancreas does not produce enough insulin or when the body cannot effectively use the insulin produced. There are two basic forms of diabetes: type 1 and type 2. People with type 1 diabetes do not produce enough insulin. People with type 2 diabetes produce insulin but cannot use it effectively.

Diabetic foot: A foot that exhibits any pathology that results directly from diabetes or complications of diabetes.

Diabetic ketoacidosis (DKA): DKA happens when there is not enough insulin and cells become starved for sugars. An alternative source of energy called ketones becomes activated. The system creates a build-up of acids and can lead to coma and even death.

Epidemiology: The study of the occurrence and distribution of health-related states or events in specific populations, including the study of the determinants influencing such states, and the applications of this knowledge to the control of health problems.

Fats: Substances that help the body utilise some vitamins and help keep the skin healthy. They are also the main way the body stores energy. In food there are many types of fats: saturated, unsaturated, polyunsaturated, monounsaturated and trans fats.

Fructose: A type of sugar found in many fruits and vegetables and in honey.

Gestational diabetes mellitus (GDM): Diabetes first diagnosed during pregnancy which resolves after childbirth.

Glucagon: A hormone secreted by the pancreas; stimulates increases in blood sugar levels in the blood (thus opposing the action of insulin).

Glucose: Also called dextrose. The main sugar the body produces from proteins, fats and carbohydrates. Glucose is the major source of energy for living cells and is carried to each cell through the bloodstream. However, the cells cannot use glucose without the help of insulin.

Glycaemic index (GI): Glycaemic index is a measure of how quickly blood glucose rises after eating a particular type of food. Glucose has a glycaemic index of 100. The effects that different foods have on blood glucose levels vary considerably. The glycaemic index estimates how much each gram of available carbohydrate (total carbohydrate minus fibre) in a food raises a person's blood glucose level following consumption of the food, relative to consumption of pure glucose.

Glycogen: Glycogen is a long molecule of linked-together glucose units (polysaccharides) that acts as a form of energy storage in animals. This polysaccharide structure represents the main storage form of glucose in the body and is analogous to starch, the energy storage molecule found in plants.

In humans, glycogen is made and stored primarily in the cells of the liver and the muscles, and functions as the secondary long-term energy storage. Muscle glycogen is converted into glucose by muscle cells, and liver glycogen converts to glucose for use throughout the body. As an energy reserve, it can be quickly drawn upon to meet a sudden need for glucose.

Glycosylated haemoglobin (HbA1c): See below.

HbA1c (glycated haemoglobin test): Haemoglobin is a protein in red blood cells that comprises globin and iron-containing haem, which transports oxygen from the lungs to the tissues of the body. Glycosylated haemoglobin is haemoglobin to which glucose is chemically bound. It is tested to monitor long-term control of diabetes. The level of glycosylated haemoglobin is increased in the red blood cells of persons with poorly controlled diabetes.

Hormone: A chemical substance secreted by an endocrine gland or group of endocrine cells that acts to control or regulate specific physiological processes, including growth, metabolism, and reproduction. Most hormones are secreted by endocrine cells in one part of the body and then transported by the blood to their target site of action in another part, though some hormones act only in the region in which they are secreted.

Hyperglycaemia: A raised level of glucose in the blood, a sign that diabetes is out of control. It occurs when the body does not have enough insulin or cannot use the insulin it does have to turn glucose into energy. Signs of hyperglycaemia are of excessive thirst, dry mouth and a need to urinate often.

Hypertension: Abnormally high blood pressure, especially in the arteries. Often referred to as high blood pressure. High blood pressure increases the risk for heart attack and stroke.

Hypoglycaemia: Too low a level of glucose in the blood. This occurs when a person with diabetes has injected too much insulin, eaten too little food or has exercised without extra food. A person with hypoglycaemia may feel nervous, shaky, weak, sweaty and have a headache, blurred vision and hunger.

Impaired fasting glucose (IFG): Impaired fasting glucose is a category of higher than normal blood glucose, but below the diagnostic threshold for diabetes after fasting (typically after an overnight fast). People with IFG are at an increased risk of developing diabetes.

Impaired glucose tolerance (IGT): Impaired glucose tolerance (IGT) is a category of higher than normal blood glucose but below the diagnostic threshold for diabetes, after ingesting a standard amount of glucose in an oral glucose tolerance test. People with IGT are at an increased risk of developing diabetes.

Impotence: Also called erectile dysfunction and is a persistent inability of the penis to become erect or stay erect. Some men may become impotent after having diabetes for a long time because nerves and blood vessels to the penis become damaged.

Incidence: It indicates how often a disease occurs. More precisely, it corresponds to the number of new cases of a disease among certain groups of people for a certain period of time.

Insulin: A hormone whose main action is to enable the body cells to absorb glucose from the blood and use it as energy. Insulin is produced by the beta cells of the islets of Langerhans in the pancreas.

Insulin resistance: Insulin resistance (IR) is the condition in which cells fail to respond to the normal actions of the hormone insulin. The body produces insulin, but the cells in the body become resistant to insulin and are unable to use it as effectively, leading to hyperglycaemia. Beta cells in the pancreas subsequently increase their production of insulin.

Islets of Langerhans: Named after the German anatomist, Paul Langerhans, who discovered them in 1869, these clusters of cells are located in the pancreas and contain its endocrine (hormone-producing) cells. They make up approximately 2 per cent of the pancreas.

Nephropathy: Damage to small blood vessels in the kidney in a person with diabetes, leading to impaired kidney function.

Neuropathy: Damage to nerves due to diabetes, causing a variety of symptoms including numbness or tingling in the feet and erectile dysfunction.

Obesity: The term used to describe excess body fat. It is defined in terms of an individual's weight and height or his/her body mass index (BMI). A BMI over 30 is classified as being obese. Obesity makes your body less sensitive to insulin's action and extra body fat is thought to be a risk factor for diabetes.

Pancreas: The pancreas is a glandular organ situated behind the lower part of the stomach and contains endocrine cells that produce the critical hormones insulin and glucagon and also has a digestive role.

Protein: Proteins are one of three main types of food and are made of amino acids, which are called the building blocks of the cells. All cells need protein to grow and to repair themselves. Protein is found in many foods such as meat, fish, poultry, eggs, legumes, and dairy products.

Randomised controlled trials: These are trials designed to test whether a treatment is effective. Patients are split into groups. One group is given the treatment being tested while another group (called the comparison or control group) is given an alternative treatment, which could be a different type of drug or a dummy treatment (a placebo). The results are then compared.

Renal: Relating to the kidneys.

Retina: Part of the back lining of the eye that senses light and is fed by many small blood vessels that can be damaged by diabetes.

Retinopathy: Retinopathy is a disease of the retina of the eye, which may cause visual impairment or blindness.

Starch: Starch is a carbohydrate consisting of a large number of glucose units joined together. A polysaccharide, it is produced by most green plants as an energy store. It is the most common carbohydrate in human diets and is contained in large amounts in such staple foods as potatoes, wheat, maize (corn) and rice.

Stroke: A sudden loss of function in part of the brain as a result of the interruption of its blood supply by a blocked or burst artery.

Sulfonylureas: A type of medication that helps lower the level of sugar in the blood by stimulating the pancreas to produce more insulin.

Triglyceride: Fats carried in the blood and derived from the foods we eat. Most of the fats we eat, including butter, margarines and oils, are in triglyceride form. An excess of triglycerides is stored in fat cells throughout the body. The body needs insulin to remove this type of fat from the blood.

Type 1 diabetes: Type 1 diabetes mellitus develops most frequently in children and adolescents. About 10 per cent of people with diabetes have type 1 diabetes. The symptoms of type 1 diabetes vary in intensity and include excessive thirst, excessive passing of urine, weight loss and lack of energy. Insulin is a life-sustaining medication for people with type 1 diabetes and they require daily injections for survival.

Type 2 diabetes: Type 2 diabetes mellitus is much more common than type 1 diabetes and occurs mainly in adults, although it is now seen increasingly in children and adolescents. The symptoms of type 2 diabetes are usually less marked than in type 1 diabetes. Some people with type 2, however, have no early symptoms and are only diagnosed several years after the onset of the condition when various diabetic complications are already present. Recent scientific research has shown that fat deposited in the liver and pancreas may be impairing the functions of these organs and causing type 2 diabetes. Reversal (partial or complete) of the condition is now thought possible through a combination of calorie restriction and increased physical activity.

NOTES

Chapter 2: What is type 2 diabetes?

1. The UK Prospective Diabetes Study (UKPDS) was a landmark randomised, multicentre trial of glycaemic therapies in 5,102 people with newly diagnosed type 2 diabetes. It ran for 20 years (1977 to 1997) in 23 UK clinical sites and showed conclusively that the complications of type 2 diabetes, previously often regarded as inevitable, could be reduced by improving blood glucose and/or blood pressure control. The UKPDS was designed and run by the late Professor Robert Turner and Professor Rury Holman. http://www.dtu.ox.ac.uk/ukpds_trial/

Chapter 3: The complications of diabetes

1. Fact sheet about diabetic retinopathy: http://www.retinal screening.nhs.uk/userFiles/File/diabeticRetinopathyFacts. pdf

Chapter 5: The diabetes and obesity epidemic

1. Ravussen, E, Bennett PH et al., 'Effect of a Traditional Lifestyle on Obesity in Pima Indians', *Diabetes Care*, 17, (1994) 1067–1074
2. Curtis, M, 'The Obesity Epidemic in the Pacific Islands', *Journal of Development and Social Transformation*, 1, (2004), 37–42
3. *IDF Diabetes Atlas*, 6th ed., (International Diabetes Federation, 2013)
4. Matthews, DR, Matthews, PC, 'Type 2 diabetes as an infectious disease: is this the black death of the 21st century?', *Diabetes Medicine* 28, (2011), 2–9

5. Taylor, R, 'Type 2 diabetes etiology and reversibility', *Diabetes Care*, 36, (2013), 1047

Chapter 6: Can diabetes be reversed?

1. Diabetes Prevention Program Research Group, 'Reduction in the incidence of type 2 diabetes with lifestyle intervention or metformin', *New England Journal of Medicine*, 346, (2002) 393–403

2. Lindstrom, J, Erikkson J, Louheranta A et al., 'The Finnish diabetes prevention study (DPS)', *Diabetes Care*, 26 (2003), 3230–3236

3. James, J, Thomas, P, Cavan DA, Kerr D et al., 'Preventing childhood obesity by reducing consumption of carbonated drinks: cluster randomised controlled trial', *British Medical Journal*, 328, (2004), 1237

4. Franco, M, Bilal, U, Ordumez P et al., 'Population-wide weight loss and regain in relation to diabetes burden and cardiovascular mortality in Cuba 1980–2010: repeated cross sectional surveys and ecological comparison of secular trends', *BMJ*, 346, (2013), f1515, doi: 10.1136/bmj.f1515

5. Guidone, C, Manco, M et al., 'Mechanisms of recovery from type 2 diabetes after malabsorptive bariatric surgery', *Diabetes*, 55, (2006)

6. Lim, EL, Hollingsworth, KG, Taylor, E et al., 'Reversal of type 2 diabetes: normalisation of beta cell function in association with decreased pancreas and liver triacylglycerol', *Diabetologia*, 54, (2011), 2506–2514

7. Steven, E, Lim, L, Taylor, R, 'Population response to information on reversibility of Type 2 diabetes', *Diabetic Medicine*, 30, (2013), e135–e138

8. Gregg, EW, Chen, H et al., 'Association of an intensive lifestyle intervention with remission of type 2 diabetes', *Journal of the American Medical Association*, 308, (2012), 2489–96, doi: 10.1001/jama.2012.67929

Chapter 7: The importance of losing weight

1. Mosley, M, *The Fast Diet: The Secret of Intermittent Fasting: Lose Weight, Stay Healthy, Live Longer*, (Short Books. 2013)

Chapter 8: Why we eat what we eat

1. Briffa, J, *Escape the Diet Trap*, (Fourth Estate, 2013)

Chapter 9: All about carbohydrates

1. Eight tips for health eating. http://www.nhs.uk/Livewell/Goodfood/Pages/eight-tips-healthy-eating.aspx
2. Schulze, MB, Manson, JE et al., 'Sugar-sweetened beverages, weight gain, and incidence of type 2 diabetes in young and middle-aged women', *JAMA*, 292, (2004) 927–34
3. The InterAct consortium, 'Consumption of sweet beverages and type 2 diabetes incidence in European adults: results from EPIC-InterAct', *Diabetologia*, 56 (2013),1520–30
4. Gorana, MI, Ulijaszek, SJ, Ventura, EE, 'High fructose corn syrup and diabetes prevalence: A global perspective', *Global Public Health*, (2012), doi: 10.1080/17441692.2012.73625
5. Lustig, RH, 'Fructose: metabolic, hedonic, and societal parallels with ethanol', *Journal of the American Dietetic Association*, (2010)
6. Basu, S, Yoffe, P et al., 'The relationship of sugar to population-level diabetes prevalence: an econometric analysis of repeated cross sectional data', *PLoS ONE*, 8, (2013), e57873, doi:10.1371/journal.pone.0057873
7. Hu, EA, Pan, A et al., 'White rice consumption and risk of type 2 diabetes: meta-analysis and systematic review', *BMJ*, 344, (2012), e1454, doi: 10.1136/bmj.e1454 (published 16 March 2012)
8. Santos, FL, Esteves, SS et al., 'Systemic review and meta-analysis of clinical trials of the effects of low carbohydrate diets on cardiovascular risk factors', *Obesity Reviews*, 13, (2012), 1048–1066

9. Shai, I, Schwarzfuchs, D et al., 'Dietary intervention randomized controlled trial (DIRECT) group. Weight loss with a low-carbohydrate, Mediterranean, or low-fat diet', *N Engl J Med*, 359, (2008), 229–241, doi: 10.1056/ NEJMoa0708681

10. Ziaee, A, Afaghi, M et al., 'Effect of low-glycemic load diet on changes in cardiovascular risk factors in poorly controlled diabetic patients. *Indian Journal of Endocrinology and Metabolism*, 16, (2012) 991–995

11. Bozzetto, L, Prinster, A et al., 'Liver fat is reduced by an isoenergetic MUFA diet in a controlled randomized study in type 2 diabetic patients', *Diabetes Care*, (2012)

12. Sasakabe, T, Haimoto, H et al., 'Effects of a moderate low-carbohydrate diet on preferential abdominal fat loss and cardiovascular risk factors in patients with type 2 diabetes', *Journal of Diabetes, Metabolic Syndrome and Obesity*, 4, (2011), 167–174, doi: 10.2147/DMSO.S19635)

13. Jürgen E Müller, J, Dagmar Sträter-Müller, D et al., 'Carbohydrate restricted diet in conjunction with metformin and liraglutide is an effective treatment in patients with deteriorated type 2 diabetes mellitus: Proof-of-concept study', *Nutrition & Metabolism*, 8, (2011), 92

14. Cheyette, C, Balolia, Y, *Carbs & Cals*, 5th edition, (Chello Publishing, 2013)

Chapter 10: Other food types and drink

1. Estruch R, Ros, E, Salas-Salvado, J et al., 'Primary prevention of cardiovascular disease with a Mediterranean diet', *N Engl J Med*, 368, (2013), 1279–1290

2. The official five-a-day advice: http://www.nhs.uk/ Livewell/5ADAY/Pages/Why5ADAY.aspx

3. 'Is your fruit smoothie as healthy as you think?' *Which*, 15 Dec 2012 http://www.which.co.uk/news/2012/12/is-your-fruit-smoothie-as-healthy-as-you-think-305688/

4. Edmonds, CJ, Burford, D, 'Should children drink more water?', *Appetite*, 52, (2009), 776–779

5. Keijzers, GB, Bastiaan E et al., 'Caffeine can decrease insulin sensitivity in humans', *Diabetes Care*, (2002)

Chapter 11: Minerals, vitamins and supplements

1. https://www.patrickholford.com/advice/why-chromium-is-good-news
2. Balk, E et al., 'Effect of chromium supplementation on glucose metabolism and lipids: A systematic review of randomized controlled trials', *Diabetes Care*, 30, (2007), 2154–63
3. Khan, A, Safdar, M et al., 'Cinnamon improves glucose and lipids of people with type 2 diabetes', *Diabetes Care*, 26, (2003)
4. Ranasinghe, P, Jayawardana, R et al., 'Efficacy and safety of "true" cinnamon (*Cinnamomum zeylanicum*) as a pharmaceutical agent in diabetes: a systematic review and meta-analysis', *Diabetic Medicine*, (2012)
5. Talaei, A, Mohamadi, M, and Adgi, Z, 'The effect of vitamin D on insulin resistance in patients with type 2 diabetes', *Diabetology and Metabolic Syndrome*, (2013)

Chapter 12: It's time to get more active

1. Snowling, NJ, Hopkins, WG, 'Effects of different modes of exercise training on glucose control and risk factors for complications in type 2 diabetic patients', *Diabetes Care*, 29, (2006) 2518–2527
2. Umpierre, D, Ribiero, PAB, Kramer, CK et al., 'Physical activity advice only or structured exercise training and association with HbA1c levels in type 2 diabetes', *JAMA*, 305, (2011), 1790–1799
3. Andrews, RC, Cooper, AR, Montgomery, AA et al., 'Diet or diet plus physical activity versus usual care in patients with newly diagnosed type 2 diabetes: the Early ACTID randomised control trial', *Lancet*, 378, (2011); 378: 129–139
4. Morris JN, Heady JA et al., 'Coronary heart disease and physical activity at work', *Lancet*, ii (1953), 1053–1057

5. Olsen, RH et al., 'Metabolic responses to reduced daily steps in healthy nonexercising men (Reprinted)', *JAMA*, 299, (2008), 1261

6. Healy, GN., Dunstan, DW et al., 'Breaks in sedentary time: Beneficial associations with metabolic risk', *Diabetes Care*, 31, (2008)

7. Grøntved, A, Hu, FB, 'Television viewing and risk of type 2 diabetes, cardiovascular disease, and all-cause mortality: a meta-analysis', *JAMA*, 305, (2011)

8. Otten, JJ, Jones, KE et al., 'Effects of television viewing reduction on energy intake and expenditure in overweight and obese adults', *Archives of Internal Medicine*, 169, (2009)

9. Owen, N, Healy, G et al., 'Too much sitting: the population-health science of sedentary Behavior', *Exercise and Sports Science Review*

10. Cooper, R, S. Sebire, S et al., 'Sedentary time, breaks in sedentary time and metabolic variables in people with newly diagnosed type 2 diabetes', *Diabetologia*, 55, (2012), 589–599, doi: 10.1007/s00125-011-2408-x

11. Laverty et al., 'Active travel to work and cardiovascular risk factors in the United Kingdom', *American Journal of Preventative Medicine*, (2013)

12. This simple mantra was developed by Bernie Shrosbree, a former conditioning coach for the GB Olympic Rowing team who is now working with the Red Bull F1 team. It is taken from his book, *Inspired: The Blueprint for Total Conditioning*, (Hayden Publishing, 2004), which is a superb introduction to all round fitness training suitable for most people

13. Dr Michael Moseley. *Fast Exercise*, Short Books Ltd, 2013

Chapter 13: Appropriate blood glucose monitoring

1. O'Kane, MJ et al., 'Efficacy of self-monitoring of blood glucose in patients with newly diagnosed type 2 diabetes (ESMON study): randomized controlled trial', *BMJ*, (2008)

2. Ingleby, J, Trowbridge, S et al., 'Good control on blood test a week', *Diabet Med*, 19, (2002), 75

3. Franciosi, M, Lucisano, G, Pellegrini F, et al., 'ROSES: Role of self-monitoring of blood glucose and intensive education in patients with type 2 diabetes not receiving insulin: a pilot randomised clinical trial', *Diabetic Med*, 28, (2011), 789–796

4. Polonsky, WH, Fisher, L, Schikman, CH et al., 'Structured self-monitoring of blood glucose significantly reduces A1C levels in poorly controlled, noninsulin-treated type 2 patients: results from the structured testing program study', *Diabetes Care*, 34, (2011), 262–267

Chapter 14: The appropriate use of medication

1. Statistics on Obesity, Physical Activity and Diet: England, 2013. NHS: The Health and Social Care Information Centre, (2013)

2. Cohen, D, 'Rosiglitazone: what went wrong?', *BMJ*, 341, (2010) c4848

3. 'Safety alert over diabetes drug linked to bladder cancer after it is suspended in France and Germany', *Daily Mail*, 14 June 2011, http://www.dailymail.co.uk/health/article-2003149/ Safety-alert-diabetes-drug-linked-bladder-cancer-suspended-France-Germany.html#ixzz36VHg4zA7

4. More broken bones with Actos, Avandia http://www.webmd. com/diabetes/news/20080428/more-broken-bones-with-actos-avandia

5. Cohen, D, 'Has pancreatic damage from glucagon suppressing diabetes drugs been underplayed?', *BMJ*, (2013)

6. Merovci, A, Solis-Herrera, GD, Eldor, R et al., 'Dapagliflozin improves muscle insulin sensitivity but enhances endogenous glucose production', *Journal of Clinical Investigation*, 124, (2014), 509–514

Chapter 15: Managing when other illnesses strike

1. List of medications which can affect blood glucose levels. http://www.nps.org.au/conditions/hormones-metabolism-and-nutritional-problems/diabetes-type-2/for-individuals/

medicines-and-treatments/medicines-that-affect-blood-glucose-levels

Chapter 17: The importance of other health checks: the eyes, feet and kidneys

1. Information about retinal screening: http://diabeticeye.screening.nhs.uk/diabetic-retinopathy
2. Information about care planning: http://www.diabetes.org.uk/care-planning

Chapter 18: Stop smoking

1. Brown, J, Ceard, E et al., 'Real-world effectiveness of e-cigarettes when used to aid smoking cessation: a cross-sectional population study', *Addiction*, (2014), doi: 10.11111/add.12623
2. Benefits of stopping smoking: http://www.lung.ca/protect-protegez/tobacco-tabagisme/quitting-cesser/benefits-bienfaits_e.php#ref

Chapter 19: Getting support and education

1. National Service Framework for Diabetes: Standards. Department of Health 2001 https://www.gov.uk/government/publications/national-service-framework-diabetes
2. The X-pert programme: http://www.xperthealth.org.uk
3. Davies, MJ et al., 'Effectiveness of the diabetes education and self-management for ongoing and newly diagnosed (DESMOND) programme for people with newly diagnosed Type 2 diabetes: cluster randomised controlled trial', *BMJ*, 336, (2008), 491–495, http://www.desmond-project.org.uk
4. Kerr, D, Knott, J, Cavan, D, 'The changing shape of diabetes', *Practical Diabetes International*, 24 (2007),13–14
5. The eatwell plate. http://www.nhs.uk/Livewell/Goodfood/Pages/eatwell-plate.aspx

6. Trento, M, Gamba, S, Gentile, L, 'Rethink Organization to iMprove Education and Outcomes (ROMEO): A multicenter randomized trial of lifestyle intervention by group care to manage type 2 diabetes', *Diabetes Care*, 33, (2010), 745–747

Chapter 20: Reversing diabetes distress

1. Reddy, J, Wilhelm, K, Campbell, L, 'Putting PAID to diabetes-related distress: the potential utility of the problem areas in diabetes (PAID) scale in patients with diabetes', *Psychosomatics*, 54, (2013), 44–51

2. The DAWN study. http://www.dawnstudy.com/DAWN2/dawn2.asp

3. Polonsky, WH, Fisher, L et al., 'Are patients' initial experiences at the diagnosis of type 2 diabetes associated with attitudes and self-management over time?', *Diabetes Educator*, 36, (2010), 828–34

4. 'Emotional and psychological support and care in diabetes', Diabetes UK, (2010), https://www.diabetes.org.uk/Documents/Reports/Emotional_and_Psychological_Support_and_Care_in_Diabetes_2010.pdf

5. Trigwell, P et al., 'Minding the gap: the provision of psychological support and care for people with diabetes in the UK', Diabetes UK, (2008)http://www.diabetes.org.uk/Documents/Reports/Minding_the_Gap_psychological_report.pdf

INDEX

Get support from the UK's largest diabetes community

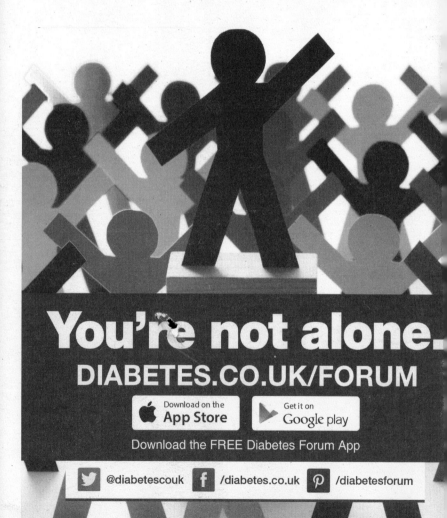